BACKYARD
MEDICINE
FOR ALL

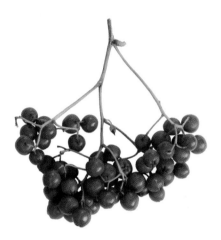

Illustrations: *above*: rowan berries; *overleaf*: a spring
harvest of primroses; *title page*: primrose leaf and
flower; *copyright page*: meadow cranesbill

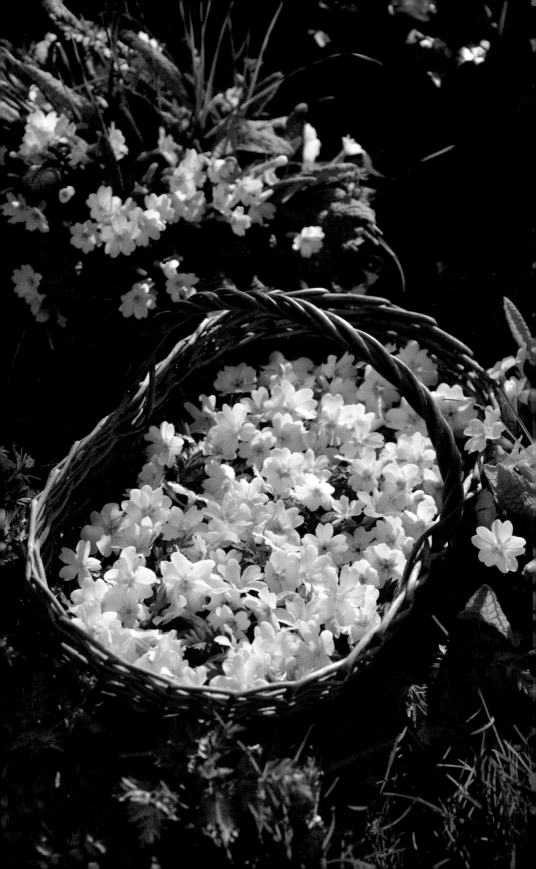

BACKYARD MEDICINE FOR ALL

A Guide to Home-Grown Herbal Remedies

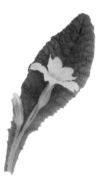

JULIE BRUTON-SEAL
MATTHEW SEAL

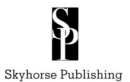

Skyhorse Publishing

Also by the Authors

Backyard Medicine

The Herbalist's Bible

Skyhorse Publishing books may be purchased in bulk at special discounts for sales promotion, corporate gifts, fund-raising, or educational purposes. Special editions can also be created to specifications. For details, contact the Special Sales Department, Skyhorse Publishing, 307 West 36th Street, 11th Floor, New York, NY 10018 or info@skyhorsepublishing.com.

Skyhorse® and Skyhorse Publishing® are registered trademarks of Skyhorse Publishing, Inc.®, a Delaware corporation.

Visit our website at www.skyhorsepublishing.com.

10 9 8 7 6 5 4 3 2 1

Library of Congress Cataloging-in-Publication Data is available on file.

Cover design by Adam Bozarth

Print ISBN: 978-1-5107-2594-2
Ebook ISBN: 978-1-5107-2595-9

Printed in China

Contents

To the plants and all our other teachers

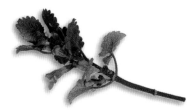

Country people heretofore did often use [ground ivy, above] to tun
it up with their drink…. But this Age forsakes all old things, though
never so good, and embraceth all kind of novelties whatsoever; but
the time will come, that the fopperies of the present time shall be
slighted, and the true and honest prescriptions of the Ancients come
in request again.
– William Coles (1656)*

Rather than dismissing items of plant lore as quaint reminders of
a more ignorant past, they should be seen as clues to an earlier, far
more comprehensive knowledge of the use of plants.
– Gabrielle Hatfield (1999)

* For all references and sources, see Notes to the Text, starting on p214

Preface

We wrote this book because we saw around us a wealth of plants growing abundantly, which have medicinal uses that people have largely forgotten. These plants were once valued and widely used, but over time fell out of fashion and were bypassed because of a focus on the herbs of commerce.

Many readers of our earlier book *Hedgerow Medicine* have noted our hint there that we had another 50 or more plants in mind for similar treatment. In *Backyard Medicine for All* we have made room for these and a few more, including cognate species in a single chapter – such as primrose and cowslip; silverweed, tormentil and cinquefoil – or family groups, eg cranesbills, speedwells and thistles.

This is in effect a sequel to *Hedgerow Medicine*, with a similar locale and rationale. It has the same layout, with its strong visual emphasis, and the same sequence of information. As the subtitle suggests, we focus on largely forgotten medicinal plants that grow by roads or paths in the countryside or in the city.

Wayside plant medicine may start for you with reading a book like this, but the aim is for you to go out and practise it. Even Mr Squeers, the almost-illiterate headmaster in Dickens' *Nicholas Nickleby*, would agree. On Nicholas' first day at school, Squeers says:

"When the boys knows this out of book, he goes and does it. Where's the second boy?"
"Please, sir, he's weeding the garden."
"To be sure. So he is. B-O-T, bot, T-I-N, bottin, N-E-Y, bottiney, noun substantive, a knowledge of plants. When he has learned that bottiney means a knowledge of plants, he goes and knows 'em. That's our method, Nickleby.
"Third boy, what's a horse?"

And where do we 'go and know' for our practical lessons? To what the late Roger Deakin called *the undiscovered country of the nearby*. Waysides of old have become the road verges of today, and these everyday, nearby but overlooked ecosystems are significant wild plant communities.

Each chapter has an introductory section that puts the plant(s) into historical and botanical context, and its forgotten or traditional medicinal uses; the Use For section describes current medicinal applications; and a new final section, Modern Research, selects from published clinical work about the plant (mainly from the PubMed database). We dislike animal studies for several reasons but have included some as they can inspire further exploration.

The medicinal recipes have an important role. We subscribe to the advice of noted herbalist Christopher Hedley: *Don't buy a herbal book if it doesn't have recipes!* Making a medicine from it is the ultimate relationship with a plant, and we hope you will move from the armchair to the roadside, with due cautions noted, and try these recipes for yourself.

But, why 'forgotten' plants? Mostly these are plants that were once in the herbal pharmacopoeia but have been dropped as chemical medicines replaced them, and as the pharmacopoeias themselves shrank. Once out of the 'official' lists, plants are no longer commercially attractive and disappear from everyday use and familiarity.

Herbal knowledge has been declining since a peak in the mid-17th century, when John Parkinson included some 3,800 herbs in his great herbal. But we can do something about it. Contemporary American herbalist David

Winston, writing in 2005, made a plea that we heartily endorse: *One way of correcting this problem is the expansion of our pharmacopoeias by the inclusion of unused but effective indigenous and introduced species. There are hundreds of such herbs available that have long histories of usage by peoples who depended on these plants for their health and well being.*

Winston offers about a hundred plants for an 'American extra pharmacopoeia'. Indeed, several of them overlap with our choices (eg chicory, cow parsnip/hogweed, ground ivy, ox-eye daisy and purple loosestrife).

What are our rules for a plant's inclusion in this book? We cover plants we have had experience of; local abundance on waysides (eg navelwort is common in the west but not otherwise in the UK); we wanted to include juniper and centaury but they are endangered in the wild, so we didn't; ease of identification; being non-poisonous (eg we explain at length how other Apiaceae species differ from hemlock); and above-ground parts rather than roots.

Harvest with respect is our belief, so don't pick more than you need even where a row of hogweed stretches to the horizon along your roadside. It will be there tomorrow, unless the council mower happens to pass by.

Writing a book like this is a collaborative process, not only between ourselves as co-authors but also within a wider herbal community. Our heartfelt thanks go to: Julian Barker, Charlotte du Cann, Danny O'Rawe and Mark Watson for acting as expert sounding boards in our contents-selection process; to Julia Behrens, Alice Bettany, Andrew Chevallier, Nikki Darrell, Chris Gambatese, Barbara Griggs, Karin Haile, Simon Harrap, Glennie Kindred, 7Song, Cathy Skipper and Davina Wynne-Jones for herbal wisdom, freely shared; and to Christine Herbert for (as usual) reading

every word and offering us acute comments – and letting us photograph or pick plants in her smallholding. We also thank the Forgotten Herbs Facebook group, and forager friends Mina Said-Allsopp, Robin Harford and Monica Wilde.

To Merlin Unwin, Karen McCall and Jo Potter of Merlin Unwin Books our renewed thanks for getting the carrot/stick ratio just right.

We are grateful to a number of institutions, including the Wellcome Library, the British Library and the Norfolk County Council library service. We especially thank our local bibliographic treasure-house, the John Innes Historical Collections and outreach curator Dr Sarah Wilmot.

We have acknowledged sources in the Notes to the Text, and thank copyright holders for permission to include extracts from their work. If we have overlooked or been unable to locate copyright owners we will gladly add details in a later edition. Needless to say, the opinions expressed here are our own, and we take responsibility for them.

Thanks also to Julie's many patients who, wittingly or not, have contributed to this book. Don't worry, you remain anonymous.

Finally, our respect to the plants themselves. We owe them everything, for, as John Ruskin wrote over 150 years ago:

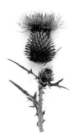

All the wide world of vegetation blooms and buds for you; the thorn and the thistle which the earth casts forth as evil are to you the kindliest servants; no dying petal nor drooping tendril is so feeble as to have no help for you.

Julie Bruton-Seal & Matthew Seal
Ashwellthorpe, Norfolk
November 2016

Introduction

Jesus' Parable of the Sower starts with the seeds that fall by the wayside – *and the fowls came and devoured them up* (Matthew 13.4). This wayside is hard and impenetrable, unsuitable ground for hand-spread seeds to germinate. In effect they were bird food.

The parable next has seeds falling on stony ground, which grew but scorched in the sun because they had no root. Seed scattered on thorny ground germinated but was choked by weeds. The seed on fertile ground flourished, and gave varying levels of fruit.

The parable explains different levels of faith. But what concerns us here is an undertone: in the battle of agriculture and nature, cultivated crops must win against weeds, or we all die. 'Falling by the wayside' is a metaphor for losing out, giving up and being forgotten, as morally inferior. Waysides are marginal land, between public road and private farmland, lacking the status and value of either.

Yet European and other pre-industrial waysides were once vibrant spaces, tracks where multitudes of people and livestock moved between fields and villages, while ancient droveways saw cattle led hundreds of miles to distant urban markets. Carts and carriages used animal power, and as draught horses or cows grazed the wayside vegetation they also fertilised it. It was a wayside golden age for wild flowers where meadows met mud tracks, and grass was kept short.

Fast forward to today, and livestock is moved by truck, people drive rather than walk, fields are over-fertilised, roads are metalled over, mass levels of traffic emit nitrous oxide pollutants, and hedges and roadsides are cut by mowers owned by councils or landowners. The wayside wild plants are often mown in early summer, when all but spring plants have yet to complete their life cycle, and the sward is left uncollected, leading to excess nitrogenous content in the soil. This favours nitrogen-loving summer species like hogweed (cow parsnip), nettle and bramble, which choke other plants – thorny ground indeed.

The plant conservation charity Plantlife estimates that 97% of British meadows have gone since the 1930s. No wonder that the few remaining animal-based rural economies in places like parts of Romania, Sardinia, Poland or Amish lands in Pennsylvania are celebrated, a reminder of the lost wealth of ancient meadowlands and waysides.

Yet all is not a forgotten memory. Plantlife estimates that about 700 species of wild plants still grow on Britain's road verges, some 45% of the nation's flora. And there are nearly 320,000 miles (500,000 km) of these verges. They are effectively the residual habitat of lost meadows, and they are already managed. And sometimes protected: we live near Wood Lane Road-verge Meadow, Long Stratton, home of the endangered sulphur clover.

Taking 'road-verge' as the modern equivalent of 'way-side' opens everything up. Why not locate and use some of these abundant, free, easily identified (in most cases) and wiry wild wayside plants for our own medicine? This book invites you to step off the 'beaten track' and offers you the means to do so, including the legalities and practicalities of collecting wayside plants for medicinal use.

Harvesting from the wayside

Harvesting wild plants for food or medicine is a great pleasure, and healing in its own right. We all need the company of plants and wild places, whether a wayside, an old wood, a remote moor or seashore or even our own garden. Gathering herbs for free is the beginning of a valuable and therapeutic relationship with the wild. Here are a few basic guidelines to get started.

Why pay others to frolic in the luscious gardens of Earth, picking flowers and enjoying themselves making herbal products? You can do all that frolicking, immersing yourself in wondrous herbal beauty, and uplifting your mind and spirit. Making your own herbal medicine both enhances your happiness and boosts your immune system.
– Green (2000)

Herbs are to be gathered when they are fullest of juice which is before they run up to seed; and if you gather them in a hot sunshine, they will not be so subject to putrifie: the best way to dry them is in the Sun ... Let Flowers be gathered when they are in their prime, in a sunshine day, and dried in the Sun. Let the Seeds be perfectly ripe before they be gathered. Let them be kept in a dry place; for any moisture, though it be but a moist air, corrupts them.
– Culpeper (1653)

The process of gathering wild herbs for medicine – our own term for this is medicinal foraging – is straightforward. You identify the right plant and pick it at the right time, then make a simple home medicine. The benefits are aptly expressed by James Green (quote alongside), and the desiderata have not changed in the 350-plus years since Nicholas Culpeper gave his advice (below left).

Identification
Perhaps the most important thing is to ensure you have the right plant. A good field guide is essential – we like *Harrap's Wild Flowers* by Simon Harrap – and there are numerous phone apps for wild plants. A herb mentor is invaluable: many herbalists offer herb walks. Check our Resources page (220) to contact practitioners in your area.

For distribution maps and plant identification, the Botanical Society of the British Isles has a regularly updated site: see www.bsbi.org. In America the USDA maps both wild plants and crops (www.usda.gov).

Where to collect
Choose a place where the plant you are harvesting is abundant and vibrant. Woods, fields and minor roads are best, though some of our

plants are also found in the city. Avoiding heavy traffic is safer for you and your lungs, and plants growing in quiet places are less polluted. Park carefully and be aware of traffic at all times.

Remember that hedgerows next to fields may receive crop sprays and waysides may be sprayed, as well as being mown (often just when you are ready to collect).

When to collect
Harvest herbs when they are at their lushest. Pick on a dry day, after any morning dew has burned off. For aromatic plants the sun's energy is vital, so wait for a hot day and pick while the sun is high, ideally just before noon.

Harvest only what you need and will use; leave some of the plant so it will grow back. When picking above-ground parts of a plant, only take the top half to two-thirds. Never harvest if a plant is the only one in a particular area.

Collecting equipment
Very basic: think carrier bags or a basket, and perhaps gloves, hat, scissors or secateurs. Be sensible: blackthorn and sea buckthorn call for more protection than veronica. Be aware that carrying a knife with

A quiet wooded lane in
Oxfordshire, September

a blade of more than 75mm long may be a legal offence. If you are harvesting roots take a small shovel or digging fork.

We have included a few roots in our recipes. It is important not to over-harvest these, as you are usually killing the plant (exceptions include ground elder). The roots we have selected are widespread and often classed as weeds.

Collecting for sale

This book describes medicinal foraging for personal use rather than collecting for sale, either directly as in fungi to a restaurant or for making medicines or cosmetics to sell. Other laws and regulations apply when selling is involved, including health and safety approval of your equipment.

We do however like the story of Dr Christopher (1909–83), the American naturopath and herbalist, who in the lean post-war years worked as a gardener in the mornings. He kept the 'weeds' he had unearthed, notably plantain, took them home and made medicine from them. Then he sold this back to his clients!

Legal guidance

Custom in the form of common law still protects the right to wild-gather the 'four Fs' of fruit, foliage, fungi and flowers, for personal use and not resale. Roots are somewhat different, as the law recognises: it's one thing to smell a neighbour's rose, another to pick its petals and yet another to dig it up without permission.

In practical terms you should seek an owner's permission before unearthing roots anywhere outside your own garden, but picking above-ground parts of plants anywhere will generally be condoned if done discreetly and moderately. There are seldom prosecutions for medicinal harvesting.

Note that private land should be marked with a notice board, and you can theoretically be charged with trespass if you ignore such a notice. Waysides may be owned privately or be public land. Many nature reserves prohibit any picking.

Rare plants are protected by the Wildlife and Countryside Act 1981, and a list of these plants is regularly updated. No such plants are included in this book, and we would not expect to make medicine from an endangered species.

Note that legislation differs in Scotland and Scandinavian countries, with more 'right to roam' embedded in law than in England and Wales. For the text of relevant legislation, see www.legislation.gov. uk.

Storing your plants

It's a good idea to make your medicines on the same day as you pick them, if you can. And the best way to store your plants is in the medicinal form you have made, whether preserving in alcohol or glycerine, honey, vinegar, ghee, as tea or ice cubes, and so on, as outlined in the next section.

Don't forget to label any container with the plant's name, date and place collected.

Using your wayside harvest

Herbs can be used in many different ways. Simplest and most ancient is nibbling the fresh plant, crushing the leaves to apply them as a poultice or perhaps boiling up some water to make a tea. Many of the plants discussed in this book are foods as well as medicines, and incorporating them seasonally in your diet is a tasty and enjoyable way to improve your health.

But because fresh herbs aren't available year round or may not grow right on your doorstep, you may want to preserve them for later use. Follow these guidelines.

Equipment needed

You don't need any special equipment for making your own foraged medicines. You probably already have most of what you need.

Kitchen basics like a teapot, measuring jugs, saucepans and a blender are all useful, as are jam-making supplies such as a jelly bag and jam jars. A mortar and pestle are handy but not essential. You'll also need jars, bottles and labels for these.

There is a list of suppliers at the end of the book to help you source any supplies or ingredients you may need (see p220).

It is a good idea to have a notebook to write down your experiences, so you'll have a record for yourself and can repeat successes. Who knows, it could become a family heirloom like the stillroom books of old!

Drying herbs

The simplest way to preserve a plant is to dry it, and then use the dried part as a tea (infusion or decoction: see overleaf). Dried plant material can also go into tinctures, infused oils and other preparations, though these are often made directly from fresh plants.

To dry herbs, tie them in small bundles and hang these from the rafters or a laundry airer, or spread the herbs on a sheet of brown paper or a screen. (Avoid using newspaper as the inks contain toxic chemicals.)

Generally, plants are best dried out of the sun. An airing or warming cupboard works well, particularly in damp weather.

You can easily make your own drying screen by stapling some mosquito netting or other open-weave fabric to a wooden frame. This is ideal, as the air can circulate around the plant, and yet you won't lose any small flowers or leaves through the mesh.

A dehydrator set on a low temperature setting is perfect for drying herbs as well as summer fruit.

Storing dried herbs

Once the plant is crisply dry, you can discard any larger stalks. Whole leaves and flowers will keep best, but if they are large you may want

The 'Virtues' of a herb are its strengths and qualities; its inner potency, expressions of its vital spirit and of the way it is in the world. The way a herb is in the world will inform it of the way to be in your body. We prefer this term to the more modern 'uses'. Herbs do not have uses. They have themselves and their own purposes.
– Hedley & Shaw (2016)

to crumble them so they take up less space. They will be easier to measure for teas etc if they are crumbled before use.

Dried herbs can be stored in brown paper bags or in airtight containers such as sweet jars or plastic tubs, in a cool place. If your container is made of clear glass or other transparent material, keep it in the dark as light will fade leaves and flowers quite quickly.

Dried herbs will usually keep for a year, until you can replace them with a fresh harvest. Roots and bark keep longer than leaves and flowers.

In looking at medicine-making we start with the familiar teas and tinctures, then move on to often-forgotten but still valuable methods.

Teas: infusions and decoctions
The simplest way to make a plant extract is with hot water. Use fresh or dried herbs. An **infusion**, where hot water is poured over the herb and left to steep for several minutes, is the usual method for a tea of leaves and flowers.

A **decoction**, where the herb is simmered or boiled in water for some time, is best for roots and bark. Decoctions stored in sterile bottles will keep for a year or more if unopened.

Infusions and decoctions can also be used as mouthwashes, gargles, eyebaths, fomentations and douches.

Tinctures
While the term tincture can refer to any liquid extract of a plant, what is usually meant is an alcohol and water extract. Many plant constituents dissolve more easily in a mixture of alcohol and water than in pure water. There is the added advantage of the alcohol being a preservative, allowing the extract to be stored for several years.

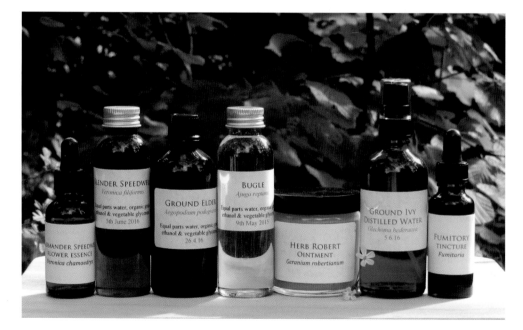

The alcohol content of the finished extract needs to be at least 20% to adequately preserve it. Most commercially produced tinctures have a minimum alcohol content of 25%. A higher concentration is needed to extract more resinous substances, such as pine resin.

For making your own tinctures, vodka is preferred as it has no flavour of its own, and allows the taste of the herbs to come through. Whisky, brandy or rum work quite well too. Wine can be used, especially for dried herbs, but will not have as long a shelf life because of its lower alcohol content.

To make a tincture, you simply fill a jar with the herb and top up with alcohol, or you can put the whole lot in the blender first. The mixture is then kept out of the light for anything from a day to a month to infuse before being strained and bottled. The extraction is ready when the plant material has lost most of its colour.

Tinctures are convenient to store and to take. We find amber or blue glass jars best for keeping, although clear bottles will let you enjoy the colours of your tinctures. Store them in a cool place. Kept properly, most tinctures have a shelf life of around five years. They are rapidly absorbed into the bloodstream, and alcohol makes the herbal preparation more heating and dispersing in its effect.

Wines and beers
Many herbs can be brewed into wines and beers, which will retain the medicinal virtues of the plants. Elderberry wine and nettle beer are traditional, but don't forget that ordinary beer is brewed with hops, a medicinal plant.

Other fermentations
There are other fermentations that use a combination of yeasts and bacteria. Sourdough bread is one example, but more relevant here are drinks such as kefir and kombucha. The starter grains are usually available on eBay.

There are two kinds of kefir, one made with milk and one made with sugar and water. We find the latter a really useful drink that can be flavoured with various herbs, such as in our sea buckthorn recipe on p160.

Glycerites
Vegetable glycerine (glycerol) is extracted from vegetable oil, and is a sweet, syrupy substance. It is particularly good in making medicines for children, and for soothing preparations intended for the throat and digestive tract, or coughs. A glycerite will keep well as long as the concentration of glycerine is at least 50% to 60% in the finished product.

Glycerine does not extract most plant constituents as well as alcohol does, but preserves flavours and colours better, and is particularly good for flowers. Glycerites are made the same way as tinctures, except the jar is kept in the sun or in a warm place to infuse.

Many herbalists like to add a small amount of alcohol to their glycerites to help preserve them, and to make them less sweet.

Glycerine is a good preservative for fresh plant juices, in which half fresh plant juice and half glycerine are mixed, as it keeps the juice green and in suspension better than alcohol. This preparation is called a succus.

Gemmotherapy extracts
Gemmotherapy is nothing to do with gem stones but rather uses the buds, shoots and sometimes root tips of trees and shrubs. The idea is that the embryonic tissue in the growing tips contains all the information of the whole plant, as well as various hormones not present elsewhere in the plant.

Buds are collected when they are plump but still firm, just before they open. Shoots are picked green, when they emerge from the dormant twigs. Because picking off the growth tip of a tree branch stops that part producing leaves, it needs to be done respectfully, not taking too many from any one plant.

For extracting the chemistry of buds and shoots, a mixture of equal parts water, alcohol and glycerine has been found most effective. If you are using vodka or another spirit that is 50% alcohol (or more usually 40% alcohol and 60% water), simply use two parts alcohol to one part glycerine.

We have found this an effective mixture for roots and leaves too, and often prefer it to making a standard tincture or glycerite.

Vinegars
Another way to extract and preserve plant material is to use vinegar. Some plant constituents will extract better in an acidic medium, making vinegar the perfect choice.

Herbal vinegars are often made from pleasant-tasting herbs, and used in salad dressings and for cooking. They are also a good addition to the bath or for rinsing hair, as the acetic acid of the vinegar helps restore the natural protective acid pH of the body's exterior. Cider vinegar is a remedy for colds and other viruses, so it is a good solvent for herbal medicines made for these conditions.

Herbal honeys
Honey has natural antibiotic and antiseptic properties, making it an excellent vehicle for medicines to fight infection. It can be applied topically to wounds, burns and leg ulcers. Local honeys can help prevent hayfever attacks.

Honey is naturally sweet, making it palatable for medicines for children. It is also particularly suited to medicines for the throat and respiratory system as it is soothing and also clears congestion. Herb-infused honeys are made the same way as glycerites.

Oxymels
An oxymel is a preparation of honey and vinegar. Oxymels were once popular as cordials, both in Middle Eastern and European herbal traditions. They are particularly good for cold and flu remedies. Honey can be added to a herb-infused vinegar, or an infused honey can be used as well.

Electuaries
These are basically herbal pastes. They are often made by stirring powdered dried herbs into honey or glycerine, but also by grinding up herbs, seeds and dried fruit together. Electuaries are good as children's remedies, soothe the digestive tract and can be made into tasty medicine balls or truffles.

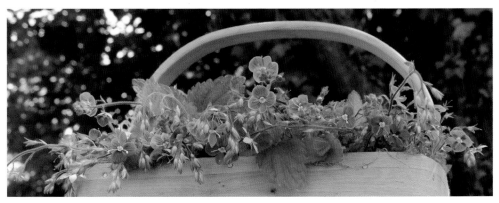

Syrups

Syrups are made by boiling the herb with sugar and water. The sugar acts as a preservative, and can help extract the plant material. Syrups generally keep well, especially the thicker ones containing more sugar, as long as they are stored in sterilised bottles.

They are particularly suitable for children because of their sweet taste, and are generally soothing.

Herbal sweets

While we are not recommending large amounts of sugar as being healthy, herbal sweets such as coltsfoot rock and peppermints are a traditional way of taking herbs in a pleasurable way.

Plant essences

Plant essences, usually flower essences, differ from other herbal preparations in that they only contain the vibrational energy of the plant, and none of the plant chemistry. They have the advantage of being potent in small doses. Julie nearly always dispenses flower essences for her patients alongside other herbal preparations as they help the herbs do their job.

To make an essence, the flowers or other plant parts are usually put in water in a glass bowl and left to infuse in the sun for a couple of hours, as in the instructions for our forget-me-not essence on p75. This essence is then preserved with brandy, and diluted for use.

Distilling herbs

While distilling essential oils from plants requires large plant quantities, it is simple to distil your own herbal waters or hydrolats.

Simply use a stockpot or other large saucepan with a domed lid that can be put on upside-down. One with a glass lid is best, as you can see what's going on inside. Put a collecting bowl in your saucepan under the centre of the lid, raised on a brick or upturned bowl above the water around it, which contains the plants. Heat the pot so that the water starts to become steam; this collects inside the lid and drips down into your collecting bowl. Ice cubes (or frozen peas!) on the upturned lid speed up the condensation. Keep on low heat until your collecting bowl is nearly full. Pour the distilled herbal water carefully into sterile bottles. There are many videos on YouTube showing you how to do this.

If you want to make larger quantities, we recommend the traditional hand-made copper alembics still being produced in Portugal. See www.al-ambiq.com

Distilled plant waters keep quite well, but do not have any preservatives, so are often dispensed in spray bottles to keep them from contamination. They are good as face washes and eyebaths, and can be taken internally. They are gentler than tinctures, but effective.

Infused oils

Oil is mostly used to extract plants for external use on the skin, but infused oils can equally well be taken internally. Like vinegars, they are good in salad dressings and in cooking.

We prefer extra virgin olive oil as a base, as it does not go rancid as many polyunsaturated oils do. Other oils, such as coconut and sesame, may be chosen because of their individual characteristics.

Infused oils are also known as macerated oils, and should not be confused with essential oils, which are aromatic oils isolated by distilling the plant material.

Ointments or salves

Ointments or salves are rubbed onto the skin. The simplest ointments are made by adding beeswax to an infused oil and heating until the beeswax has melted. The amount of wax needed will vary, depending on the climate or temperature in which it will be used, with more wax needed in hotter climates or weather.

Ointments made this way have a very good shelf life. They absorb well, while providing a protective layer on top of the skin.

Ointments can also be made with animal fats or hard plant fats such as cocoa butter, and with plant waxes such as candelilla.

Butters and ghees

Butter can be used instead of oil to extract herbs, and, once clarified by simmering, it keeps well without refrigeration, making a simple ointment. Clarified butter is a staple in Indian cooking and medicine, where it is called ghee. It is soothing on the skin and absorbs well, plumping up the skin. Herbal butters and ghees can also be used as food.

Skin creams

Creams are a mixture of a water-based preparation with an oil-based one, to make an emulsion. Creams are absorbed into the skin more rapidly than ointments, but have the disadvantages of being more difficult to make and of not keeping as well.

Creams are best refrigerated, and essential oils can be added to help preserve them. Creams are better than ointments for use on hot skin conditions, as they are more cooling.

Poultices

The simplest poultice is mashed fresh herb put onto the skin, as when you crush a plantain leaf and apply it to a wasp sting. Poultices can be made from fresh herb juice mixed with slippery elm powder or simply flour, or from dried herb moistened with hot water or vinegar.

Change the poultice every few hours and keep it in place with a bandage or sticking plaster.

Fomentations or compresses

A fomentation or compress is an infusion or a decoction applied externally. Simply soak a flannel or bandage in the warm or cold liquid, and apply. **Hot fomentations** are used to disperse and clear, and are good for conditions as varied as backache, joint pain, boils and acne. Note that hot fomentations need to be refreshed frequently once they cool down.

Cold fomentations can be used for cases of inflammation or for headaches. Alternating hot and cold fomentations works well for sprains and other injuries.

Embrocations or liniments

Embrocations or liniments are used in massage, with the herbs preserved in an oil or alcohol base, or a mixture of the two. Absorbed quickly through the skin, they can readily relieve muscle tension, pain and inflammation, and speed the healing of injuries.

Baths

Herbs can be added conveniently to bathwater by tying a sock or cloth full of dried or fresh herb to the hot tap as you run the bath, or by adding a few cups of an infusion or decoction. Herbal vinegars, tinctures and oils can be added to bath water, as can a few drops of essential oil.

Besides full baths, hand and foot baths are very refreshing, as are sitz or hip baths where only your bottom is in the water.

Part of the therapeutic effect of any of these baths is the fact that they make you stop and be still, something most of us do not do often enough.

Douches

Once they have cooled, herbal infusions or decoctions can be used as douches for vaginal infections or inflammation.

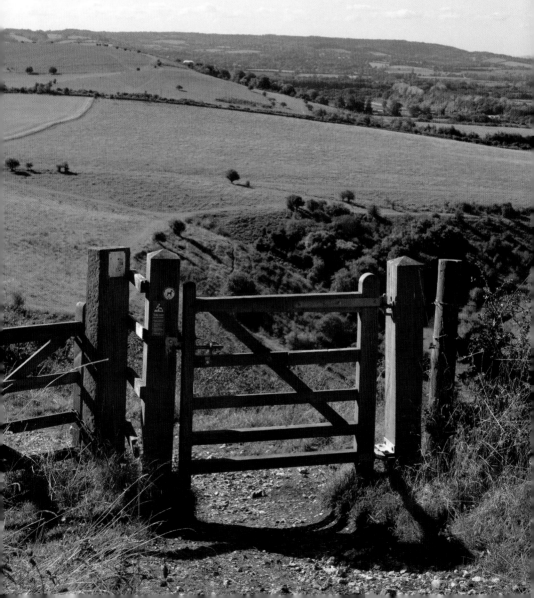

BACKYARD
MEDICINE FOR ALL

Alexanders *Smyrnium olusatrum*

Alexanders has made the switch from wild-gathered plant to cultivated and back to wild, and was both food and medicine in classical and medieval times. It lost out to celery as a commercial salad crop from the 16th century, but is now making a comeback as a winter foraged food and has intriguing possibilities in colon cancer research.

Apiaceae (Umbelliferaceae) Carrot family

Description: Tall biennial (to 1.5m or 5ft), with hairless, scented stems; leaves dark green, glossy, three-lobed; flowers yellow-white; seeds dark black ovals. Dies back in summer.

Habitat: Near the sea, by cliff and roadsides, hedgerows, forming colonies; spreading inland slowly.

Distribution: Mediterranean origin, naturalised throughout Western and Central Europe; east and southern coasts of Britain and Ireland, southern England.

Related species: Many Apiaceae are medicinal, including angelica, celery, dill, fennel and lovage. Be careful of your identification as there are several poisonous species in this family.

Parts used: All parts, including the seeds, available from autumn to spring; produces early foliage in winter.

Geoffrey Grigson (1958) says alexanders is 'happiest and most frequent by the sea'. He's right, and sturdy stands of this vigorous and stately naturalised umbellifer abound by eastern and southern coasts of Britain and Ireland.

It also seems to be pressing inland in our part of East Anglia, thriving by roadsides at least 55km (35 miles) from the Norfolk coast, perhaps responding favourably to regular winter salting of the roads.

We welcome its advance, and Julie has fond memories of picking winter alexander shoots for salad on the school run to Wroxham.

The plant's origin and names are clearly Mediterranean. Archaeological finds suggest it was being cultivated in the eastern Mediterranean in the Iron Age (c.1300–700 BC). Its roots and shoots had become a popular, if pungent, potherb and vegetable by the time of the reign of Alexander the Great in the fourth century BC.

The English name alexanders could be for the emperor, or indeed for the port in Egypt that he founded and which bore his name. The plant's Greek name *hipposelinon* means 'horse parsley or celery', which was still being used by John Parkinson in the early 17th century. In this context horse means large, according to William Salmon's herbal of 1710.

Columella, the Roman agricultural writer (AD 4–70), knew alexanders as 'myrrh of Achaea', the then current Latin name for Greece. The myrrh reference has followed the plant in its generic name *Smyrnium*. Some people do find the taste and scent to be myrrh-like, though others get more lovage in it; an old name is black lovage.

Alexanders had an early shift from wild-gathering to cultivation, and from Roman times to the 16th century or so it was more known as a food than a medicine. Its species name *olusatrum* derives from *olus* for potherb and *atrum* for black, the colour of the large seeds, which were ground as a condiment.

As both a food and medicine alexanders became a widely used monastic plant in medieval times. Many scattered inland sightings of it in Britain can be related to sites of former monastic houses. By the dissolution in the 1530s and 1540s, wild celery was being cultivated and superseded alexanders and lovage in popularity.

Currently alexanders is becoming popular again with foragers, for its fresh greens in winter and spicy seeds. We like it as a condiment to use as pepper. We actually don't find it 'peppery' but more pungent, sour, oily and nutty.

Use alexanders for ...
Alexanders was classified in classic Galenic terms as 'hot and dry in the third degree', and its actions were accordingly forceful. It was found to work strongly on the urinary and digestive systems, especially the seeds.

Parkinson (1629) states that *The seede is more used physically than the roote, or any other parte*. Salmon (1710) writes that alexanders *effectually provokes Urine, helps the Strangury, and prevails against Gravel and Tartarous Matter in Reins and Bladder*.

In modern terms, Salmon was saying that alexanders was a diuretic, clearing obstructions in the urinary system, including stones in the kidneys and bladder.

Dioscorides, in the 1st century AD, knew alexanders as an emmenagogue, a herb that promoted menstruation. Salmon noted that the plant 'powerfully provokes the Terms'; it also 'expels the Birth', ie afterbirth. That is, it is a powerful uterine tonic, to be treated with caution in pregnancy.

The Monks were good Chemists, & invented many good Receipts: which they imparted to their Penitents: & so are handed downe to their great-grandchildren, a great many varieties.
– Aubrey, c.1660s

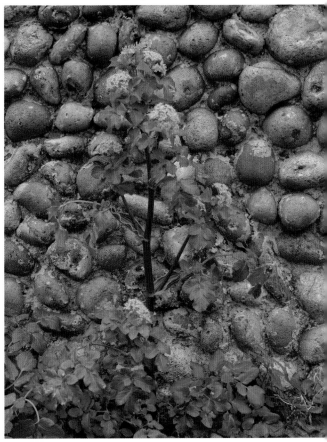

Salmon adds that a cataplasm of the bruised leaves, applied hot to the afflicted part, will dry up old sores and foetid ulcers, *and either discusses* [breaks up] *or maturates Scrophulous* [tubercular] *Tumors*.

Alexanders was included in the first London *Pharmacopoeia* (1618), meaning it was an 'official' herb of the apothecaries. But by the time Salmon prepared his herbal nearly a century later it had been dropped. It was sliding out of use in both medicine and cookery,

though there are records of alexanders root being sold to the public in Covent Garden market later in the 18th century.

Of course it does not follow that because alexanders has gone out of fashion it is no longer useful as food and a wayside medicine. The virtues the old herbalists championed remain valid, even if less used these days, and furthermore clinical experimentation is opening up some new possibilities.

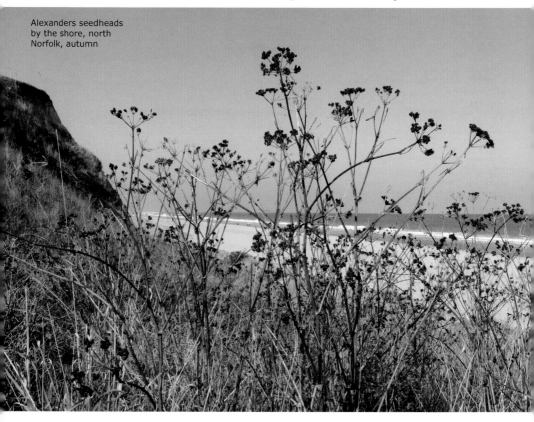

Alexanders seedheads by the shore, north Norfolk, autumn

Modern research
One area of recent interest is alexanders essential oil. Italian researchers found (2014) that the oil from the flowers induces apoptosis, or cell death, in human colon carcinoma cells. The oil has high quantities of isofuranodiene, a known anti-cancer agent.

Another intriguing finding (2012) is that this oil is strongly effective against candida, a fungal infection.

There is also a suggestion (2008) that alexanders has a comparable biomedical action to zedoary (*Curcuma wenyujin*), a type of Chinese ginger and source of a traditional remedy called Ezhu.

Ezhu is prescribed in China as an essential oil for liver, gastric, lung and cervical cancer, and its active principle, furanodiene, is the same. Perhaps alexanders could be a Western Ezhu in waiting?

Harvesting alexanders
The green herb is best harvested in winter or very early spring, before the stalks become stringy. The seeds can be harvested once they turn black, and the stems are no longer green.

A tisane for the stomak
The tisane (tea) recipe, taken from the *Syon Abbey Herbal* of 1517, may be the first English reference to alexanders as a medicinal plant (preceding the usually referenced one in William Turner's *Herball* of 1562). This quartet of four Apiaceae roots as a hot tea makes for a powerful stimulant to a sluggish stomach.

Take rotis [roots] of Fenell, Alisaundre [alexanders], Parsyly and Smalach [celery], a godehandfull, well and clen, washen and wel stanpid [crushed] in a morter & seth [boil] hem in a pottel [pot] of water to the half and do therto a littil hony and clens it and drink it at even and at moroun [morning], ix sponfull at oones [at one go].

Alexanders black butter sauce
Collect the seeds in the autumn when they are ripe. Grind them in an electric spice mill or coffee grinder. They are best freshly ground in small quantities as needed, sieving to remove any larger chunks as these can be quite chewy.

Melt 2 tablespoons **butter** with 1 tablespoon **olive oil**. Add 2 cloves **garlic**, crushed. Cook gently for a few minutes, then add 2 to 3 teaspoons **ground alexanders seeds**, and heat through.

Serve stirred into pasta, or as a dipping sauce for bread. Quite heady!

Root tisane
- sluggish digestion
- gas and griping pains
- urinary gravel
- urinary infections

Alexanders black butter sauce
- stimulates digestion
- urinary gravel

Caution
Avoid alexanders seed during pregnancy.

Ash trees in the York-
shire Dales, May

Ash *Fraxinus excelsior*

Ash has been a common British tree since Neolithic times, known as both a highly adaptable wood with a huge range of uses and as a folk medicine. It is currently in the news because it is endangered by ash dieback, a fungal disease.

Britain recognised officially in 2012 that its 126 million or so *Fraxinus excelsior* (European ash) trees were under attack by ash dieback, an almost incurable fungal condition arriving in ash trees imported from mainland Europe. The dieback manifests in the tree crowns and leaf mass, and affects saplings more readily than mature trees. Estimates in late 2015 put up to 90% of British ash trees at serious risk.

Identified first as *Chalara fraxinea*, ash dieback has been subject to intensive research, which has moved its name on twice – it is now known as *Hymenoscyphus fraxineus*. The early genome research into the fungus was carried out in the wood at the back of our house in Norfolk – and our village has the unintentionally ironic name of Ashwellthorpe.

Another threat to ash trees is the emerald ash borer, a small destructive beetle endemic to North America and now rampaging through Russia, though not found yet in the UK. It destroys a full-grown ash in three years, while *Hymenoscyphus* might take five or ten.

In cash terms, estimates say ash wood adds £100 million

Oleaceae
Olive family

Description: Grows to 30m (100ft) tall, erect, deciduous; grey bark, knobbly brown and yellow flowers, large black conical buds, bright green pinnate leaves with 7–13 oval leaflets.

Habitat: Widespread, though prefers lowland and limestone; most abundant in eastern/ southern Britain.

Distribution: Native to Northern Europe, Central and East Asia; sometimes forms woods, but also prominent in mixed woods, copses and hedgerows. Found in eastern Canada and north-eastern US.

Related species: *F. americana* (white ash); *F. angustifolia* (narrow-leaved ash); *F. chinensis* ssp. *rhynchophylla* (Chinese ash); *F. ornus* (manna ash).

Parts used: Bark, leaves, buds, fruit and seeds [keys], sap.

Here comes Betty and biochar!

The research community is not giving up on ash just yet.

In April 2016 a report by a joint British and Scandinavian team said a 200-year-old Ashwellthorpe ash tree nicknamed 'Betty' gave cause for hope.

'Betty' had three genetic markers for resisting dieback, even while living next to infected trees. The team think other British ashes share Betty's tolerance, and selective breeding may lead to resistant ash woodlands one day.

Another hopeful sign is biochar. Biochar is fine-grained charcoal made from burnt biomass, and is well known to gardeners and growers.

What is new is that enriched biochar (with added seaweed and worm casts) has lent resistance to ash dieback in an experiment in Essex, reported in 2015.

The tantalising promise is that adding biochar to ash tree roots will prevent fresh infections by fungal spores, notably those of dieback.

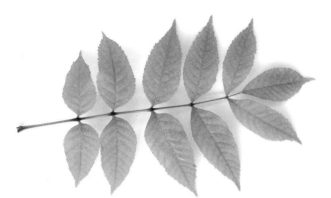

annually to Britain's economy; while ecologists remind us that ash provides a home for some 45 living species.

Even ash's glorious past has been questioned. It has long been identified as the Norse Tree of Life, Yggdrasil, with its roots in the lower world and its leaves in the heavens. But some scholars believe there has been a mistranslation, because Saga sources insist the tree is evergreen – it may be yew.

Use ash for ...

But herbal accounts offer some much-needed narrative relief. Old herbals called ash **bark** a dry bitter tonic and astringent, with anti-inflammatory and febrifuge properties. In practice this meant an ash bark decoction or tincture was drunk to clear the liver and spleen, bring down malarial fevers or ague, and also externally treat arthritis and gout.

Ash bark was often used for fevers before South American tree barks like cinchona and quinine were imported. A French herbalist calls ash *a classic family remedy for intermittent fevers as a decoction or a powder with honey.*

In Traditional Chinese Medicine (TCM) ash bark is called *Qin Pin*, with properties of clearing heat, eliminating toxins and drying internal dampness. It is used for treating diarrhoea and dysentery, and leucorrhoea.

Ash **leaves** are known as diuretic and laxative, in addition to having the properties of the bark. They were used in teas for treating gravel and small stones in the kidney, as a purgative (often combined with senna pods), and for reducing the pain of gout and water retention (dropsy). An old name for ash was gout tree.

The leaves have an old reputation as a slimming aid. William Langham wrote in 1583: *To become leane, drinke the iuice of Ash leaues now and then with wine.* Ash leaves are still included in some modern slimming formulas.

Ash **buds** have also been used for their analgesic (pain-killing) properties in arthritis and as an anti-inflammatory for relieving synovial and joint pain. The practitioners of gemmotherapy (who use spring-time buds and fresh shoots) support these uses.

Ash **fruit and seeds** (known as keys) are sometimes pickled for eating, with a caper-like taste when preserved in salt and vinegar. The keys have an ancient reputation for relieving flatulence, and as an aphrodisiac, at least in Morocco (using *F. oxyphylla*).

In French herbal tradition ash keys are *a remarkable diuretic in cases of dropsy* (Palaiseul), used in tea or powder form with honey.

The bark and leaf **sap** of some ash varieties is sweet, and known as manna. The foremost of these is *F. ornus*, the manna ash. Manna was once used as a children's laxative.

Ash is a highly versatile wood: it made arrows, wheels, tools, handles, frames and sporting accessories such as baseball bats, snooker cues and hurley sticks ('the clash of the ash' in Ireland is two hurley sticks colliding).

The writer Robert Penn (2015) tested this versatility in a novel way. He felled a large ash and commissioned craftsmen to make useful objects out of it. A year's work yielded 126 of these, with even the sawdust useful as a fuel. Ash makes excellent firewood, even when freshly cut.

Modern research
Spanish research using ash keys showed diabetes-tackling potential by lowering blood sugar levels; a wound-healing effect was demonstrated in *F. angustifolia* extracts (2015); liver fibrosis from carbon tetrachloride was reduced by *F. rhynchophylla* ethanol extracts (2010); *F. excelsior* seed had a hypoglycaemic effect in reducing blood sugars (2004).

A European Medicines Authority monograph on *F. excelsior* (2011) confined itself to confirming use of ash as a diuretic and in pain relief.

What is certain is that ash is a medicinal boon to country-dwellers.
– Palaiseul (1973)

Its fever-reducing qualities recommend it for all cases of infection, whether by virus or by bacteria. It brings down the temperature dramatically, and my father always used to refer to the ash tree as the 'quinine of Europe'.
– Mességué (1979)

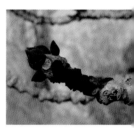
Ash buds in spring

Harvesting ash
Harvest ash leaves in summer. They can be used fresh or dried for winter use. Ash buds are gathered in spring, as they start to swell but just before they start to open.

Ash bud extract
Put your **ash buds** in a small jar. Mix enough **vodka** and **vegetable glycerine** to cover them, in the proportion of 2 parts vodka to 1 part glycerine. Leave for a month, shaking occasionally, then strain and bottle.

Dose: 10 drops three times daily

Ash leaf tea
Use one or two fresh **ash leaves**, or a rounded teaspoon of crumbled dried leaves, per mug of **boiling water**. Leave to brew for 10 to 15 minutes, then remove the leaves and drink. This tea can be drunk several times a day, as needed.

Ash bud extract
- pain
- arthritis
- joint pain

Ash leaf tea
- constipation
- urinary gravel
- gout
- dropsy
- to lose weight
- fevers
- soothes a dry throat

Avens *Geum urbanum, G. rivale*

**Roseaceae
Rose family**

Description: Wood avens *(Geum urbanum)* is a hairy perennial, to 70cm (3ft), with bright yellow flowers of 5 petals, 5 long sepals; three-part greyish leaves; a bur of brownish hooked fruits. Water avens *(G. rivale)* has beautiful, nodding purply-brown flowers.

Habitat: Wood avens is found in woodland, but is also common in gardens and hedgesides; water avens needs more moisture and shade.

Distribution: Widespread and native in British Isles, Eurasia generally. Water avens is native to US; wood avens, an introduced species to US.

Related species: Mountain avens *(Dryas octopetala)* is a rare alpine; hybrid geum *(G. x intermedium)* is a fertile cross of wood avens and water avens.

Parts used: Roots.

Where [avens] *root is in the house, the devil can do nothing, and flies from it; wherefore it is blessed above all herbs.*
– Ortus Sanitatis *(Garden of Health)* (1491)

Avens, also called wood avens or herb bennet, had a stellar medieval reputation, then retreated to more mundane uses as a potherb and moth repellant, but seems to be valued again as a rose family astringent and fever-reducing herb. Its virtues include safety, abundance and a surprising scent of cloves.

It is what lies under the earth that elevates wood avens into herb bennet, the 'blessed (*benedictus*) herb'. The name is thought to precede the lifetime of St Benedict, the monastic innovator (c.480–c.547), and refer to an older reputation that avens root would ward off evil spirits and dangerous beasts.

Avens itself is a name of uncertain origin; one supposition is that it is from the Spanish term for antidote. The genus name Geum has a more precise meaning from the Greek *geno*, to smell pleasant,

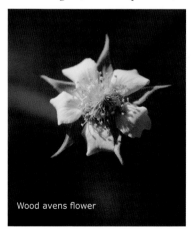

Wood avens flower

in reference to the clove-like smell of the root in spring and autumn.

It is the essential oil eugenol that gives the fragrance to avens root, as it does to cloves, nutmeg, cinnamon, basil, lemon balm and other aromatic spices and herbs. In avens itself, Polish research (2011) indicates that the time of harvest and age of the plant do not affect the amount of eugenol present.

This finding suggests that old harvesting rules of digging avens on 25 March were only partly true, and autumn roots are as potent. We have dug up the reddish-brown root of avens on several occasions, and find its smell varies in intensity according to time and place. If it doesn't smell, it could be because it is a non-fragrant hybrid geum or that the eugenol is not available; either way, it's best to return such roots to the ground.

The root is dried slowly to preserve the essential oil, and is ready when it becomes brittle. It is crushed for medicinal use, or in older times as a flavouring for a medicinal beer and wine.

Parkinson in 1640 noted: *Some use in the Spring time to put the roote to steepe for a time in wine, which giveth unto it a delicate savour and taste, which they drinke fasting every morning, to comfort the heart, and to preserve it from noisome and infectious vapours of the plague, or any poison that may annoy it.*

Avens is an antiseptic, but was not a success as a plague herb – what could be? It gradually became known as little more than a foraged potherb and broth ingredient, and a workmanlike deterrent to moths, but may be due for a herbal comeback.

Rose family astringents

We owe this category to Finnish herbalist Henriette Kress (2011). She draws attention to both the number of mild astringent herbs in the Rosaceae and the fact that they are largely interchangeable in medicinal action.

So, she writes, 'if you read that strawberry leaf works for diarrhoea, you may substitute any other astringent herb'. And, 'if you can't find anything at all, use black tea [*Camellia sinensis*, in the Theaceae], instead'. This could be a valuable guideline in your own wayside medicine-making.

Rose family astringents included in *Hedgerow Medicine* were agrimony, blackberry, hawthorn, meadowsweet, raspberry and wild rose; in this book, you will find avens, blackthorn, cinquefoil, rowan, silverweed, tormentil and wild strawberry.

Use avens for …

The description 'rose family astringent' applies to avens (see box below left). The herbalist David Hoffmann explains it well: astringents contain tannins, and in effect produce a temporary leather coat on the surface of bodily tissue. This inner surface creates a barrier to infection, and reduces irritation and inflammation.

It means that astringents as a group are good wound healers, work in the gut, relieve diarrhoea and dysentery ('bloody flux'), soothe piles and fight infection.

Avens falls into this scheme, with a specialism of combating malarial or intermittent fevers; Sir John Hill in 1812 wrote: *I have known it alone cure intermittent fevers, where the bark* [= cinchona] *has been unsuccessful.*

A common wild plant neglected, but worthy of our notice. … The root is longish and large, of a firm substance, reddish colour, and very fragrant spicy smell; it is better than many drugs kept in the shops.
– Hill (1812)

Rootstock of wood avens

Geum gee-up
- weak digestion
- poor appetite
- intermittent fevers
- convalescence
- diarrhoea

Avens mouthwash
- gum problems
- mouth ulcers

Herbalists also find avens beneficial in treatment of mouth problems, as a gargle for sore throats or an application on sore gums and mouth ulcers. The root's clove-like properties as an analgesic and antiviral help in such work, even if some 'mouth puckering' can be offputting.

The graceful water avens has similar uses, being more bitter and less aromatic (it has less eugenol in the root), and it lacks the fever-reducing benefits.

Both species are considered safe, useful remedies for everyday use.

Modern research

Polish research (2013) confirms by mass spectrometry that avens root has an essential oil and that eugenol constitutes 65–75% of it.

Romanian research (2015) gives statistical support to a posited neuroprotective activity in avens, noting a 'remarkable scavenging effect'.

More recent research (2016) proposes *G. urbanum* root as a treatment that delays α-Synuclein fibrillation in Parkinson's disease. There is no current treatment that does this.

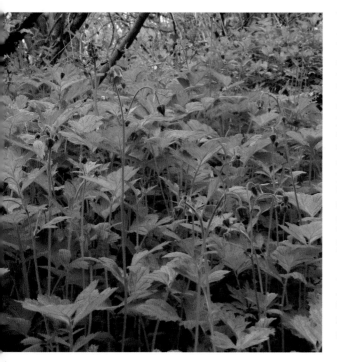

Geum gee-up

This avens root chai uses a mixture of native aromatics and hard-to-replace spices. Into a pan of boiling water add fresh (or dried) **avens roots** chopped into small pieces (your tea and cloves); add a teaspoon-size knob of **ginger**, chopped small; a teaspoon each of **alexander** seeds (for your pepper) and ripe **hogweed** seeds (for citrus/cinnamon). Add **honey** and **milk** to taste (milk optional as it's already a lovely taste) after 10 minutes. Strain. Cooled, it will keep in the fridge for up to a week.

Avens mouthwash

An avens root tea, with or without the chai ingredients, when cooled makes for an excellent mouthwash and gum rub.

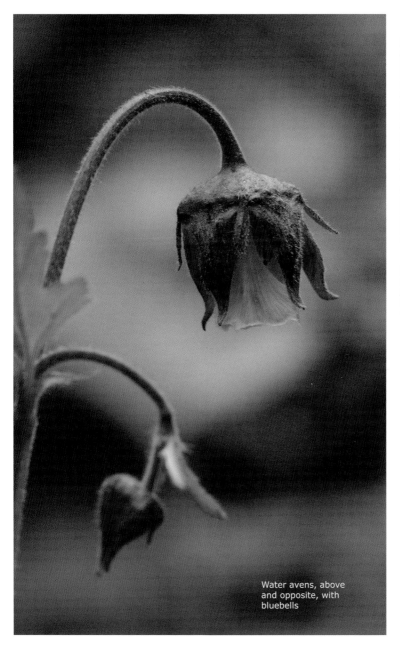

It has been said that avens is a plant that is often undervalued. There is some truth in this, for it is a sure ally against intermittent fevers, colic, diarrhoea, dysentery, circulation and liver disorders, gastric disability following acute illness, states of weakness and exhaustion, and moreover has the advantage of being easily available because it grows wild everywhere in Great Britain and Europe.
– Palaiseul (1973)

Now Geum *is fully restored in clinical practice as a safe and useful remedy.*
– Barker (2001)

Water avens, above and opposite, with bluebells

Bistort *Persicaria bistorta*

Polygonaceae
Knotweed & dock
family

Description: Large-leaved perennial native plant with prominent pink flower spikes in summer, like the fluffy boom microphones used in TV and films.

Habitat: Riverbanks, ponds, damp meadows.

Distribution: Locally abundant, mainly west and north of Britain. Also across northern Eurasia, introduced in north-eastern US.

Related species: Other common British Persicarias include redshank (*P. maculosa*), pale persicaria (*P. lapathifolia*), amphibious bistort (*P. amphibia*) and arsesmart or water-pepper (*P. hydropiper*).

Parts used: Leaves, roots.

Bistort root is one of the strongest astringent medicines in the vegetable kingdom and highly styptic and may be used to advantage for all bleedings, whether external or internal and wherever astringency is required.
– Grieve (1931)

Docks and sorrels are both in the Rumex genus within the dock family (the Polygonaceae) and embrace qualities ranging from medicinal docks to culinary sorrels. An emblematic member of the related Persicaria genus is bistort, which has an interesting history as both a spring food and as a medicine.

Bistort is named for its contorted black root, which looks 'twice twisted' (bis-tort). The S-shape also suggested a snake, leading to such other old country names as serpentary, snakeweed, adderwort and dragonwort.

Because appearance indicated purpose in a 17th-century mindset, bistort roots were presumed to be good to heal snake-bite, but there are few indications of this being effective, either in learned or folk herbal traditions.

The plant itself is communal, growing in great colonies in damp upland grassland, and its attractive pink spikes make it a popular bedding plant. Grigson (1958) found the bistort meadows *An uncommonly beautiful sight in the mountain meadows of the north,*

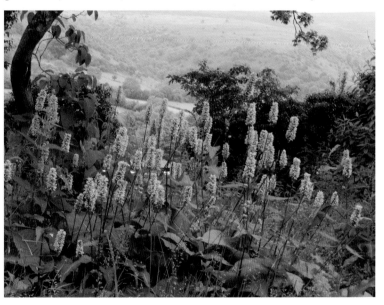

flushing the grass with pink, with spiked knaps or ears.

Bistort leaves also made for good eating as a tonic spring green. Bistort pudding was and remains food cooked in the last two weeks of Lent, hence the descriptive names of Easter mangient in Yorkshire, Easter giant in Cumberland, and passion dock in central and northern England.

Grigson proposes an interesting explanation for another name for Bistort pudding, Easter ledger or ledges. He goes back to the herbalist William Turner, who in 1548 said 'Easter ledger' was an English form of Astrologia; and Astrologia was the French name for Aristochlia or birthwort. Birthwort was an important herb in childbirth from ancient times – incidentally its other names were snakeroot or serpentary. There is

certainly an old link, weaker or stronger, with bistort as a plant of Easter and hence of new birth.

Competitive bistort pudding-making still happens each spring in the Calder valley, Yorkshire, an on-off tradition for centuries. During the Second World War, the German-supporting broadcaster 'Lord Haw Haw' (William Joyce) trumpeted that the poor Yorkshire folk had to eat grass, because they had no food. In truth they were enjoying bistort as a delicacy.

Bistort is a survival food as far afield as northern polar areas and Bangladesh. The Arctic explorer Amundsen bought bags of 'Eskimo potatoes' in the Yukon in 1905–6, probably bistort tubers, to get his team through the winter. Bistort roots are highly astringent, more so than the leaves, and could be used in tanning leather.

I found that Bistort warms and soothes the liver ... helping to dispel pressure and discomfort in that region and calming that associated feeling that one's head is going to burst with stress or frustration. ... I had mostly ignored this plant, thinking it was only good for gum problems and only had it because the supplier made a mistake!
– Blackwell (2014)

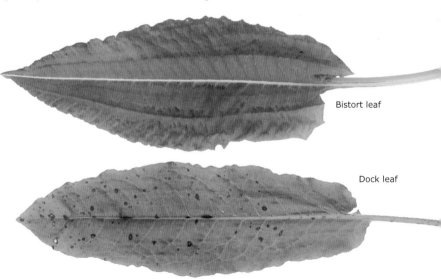

Bistort leaf

Dock leaf

Bistort, below Hardcastle Crags, Yorkshire, May. It is best as spring eating, before flowering.

Use bistort for …

The evident astringency of bistort is combined with its 'soothing demulcent' properties to make it good eating, yet also 'a gentle yet really effective plant' (Barker).

Its actions include treatments for diarrhoea, piles, ulcers, irritable bowel, mouth, gum problems and toothache (it is partly anodyne) and many types of bleeding, as visible wounds but also internally.

Modern research

Persicaria bistorta has been under-researched, but a 2014 study of the state pharmacopoeia of the Soviet Union (last edition 1990) noted that the closely related *P. maculosa* (redshanks) was 'official'. It was available in Russian pharmacies without prescription, and used as a tea for piles, as a laxative and diuretic; a tincture was taken for blood flow as an anti-coagulant.

Other Persicaria relatives of bistort have been shown by researchers to be wound-healing (2016), antioxidant (2008), anti-cancer (leukaemia) (2015) and 'potentially therapeutic' (2011) in metabolic syndrome.

This is a gentle yet really effective plant. … I find that it co-operates remarkably well with other astringents in the treatment of peptic ulcers, diverticulosis and other irritable or inflammatory conditions of the bowel providing always that chronic constipation is not present. It is the combination of soothing demulcent with tonic astringent that makes it so valuable.
– Barker (2001)

Calderdale dock (bistort) pudding
Chop two **onions** and fry gently in **butter** or oil. Coarsely chop a few handfuls of young **bistort leaves** and some young **nettle** tops, and add to the pan with a handful of **oatmeal**. Stir and cook until the leaves are tender and the oatmeal has become moistened from their juices. Season to taste with salt and pepper, and serve hot.

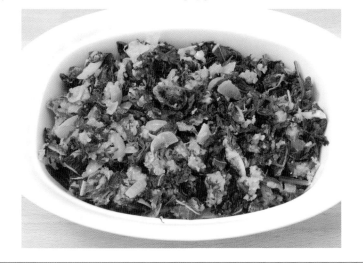

Thanks to Brenda Taylor for sharing the recipe with us: delicious!

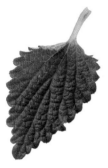

Black horehound *Ballota nigra*

A scruffy-looking wild plant, black horehound is actually an exciting 'forgotten' herb and deserves to be widely used, despite its musty smell. It is antibacterial – and notably effective against MRSA – antifungal and antiparasitic. Like its better-known cousin white horehound, it is used for coughs. It also has antispasmodic qualities and helps deal with anxiety and insomnia.

Lamiaceae
Deadnettle family

Description: A perennial to 1m (3ft) tall or more. Has a square stem, with dark and roughly hairy leaves; pinkish-purple flowers in whorls, late summer.

Habitat: Verges, waysides, walls and hedge bottoms, often on nitrogen-rich soils.

Distribution: Common in England and Wales, less frequent in Scotland and Ireland. Found across Europe to Asia and in North Africa; introduced to North and South America and New Zealand.

Related species: *B. africana*, kattekruid or kattekruie, is used in southern Africa for fevers, insomnia, piles and liver problems. *B. glandulosissima* is used similarly in Turkey.

Parts used: Flowering tops.

Eclipsed by its white horehound cousin, this plant offers valuable potential – even though its name *Ballota* comes from a Greek word meaning 'rejected', apparently because cattle refused to eat it.

White horehound (*Marrubium vulgare*) is the species more likely to be found in herb gardens, with its fuzzy white leaves, white flowers and tidier habit. A well-known cough remedy, its bitterness was sweetened by making horehound candy.

The name horehound has been given many derivations, but the most likely is from Old English *harhune*, meaning hoary or hairy plant. 'Father of English botany' William Turner (1548) had his own name for black horehound – 'stynking horehound'.

Some writers say white horehound tastes better. We disagree. Though black horehound is musty, we find it less disagreeable than the related red deadnettle or hedge woundwort, and the tincture and tea are really quite pleasant.

Black horehound tends to follow human settlement as it likes the rich nitrogenous soils found there and in places where livestock have been kept (as do elder and nettle).

One area it is appreciated is the Western Cape of South Africa and north to Namibia. The leaves are used to treat fevers and measles, and children would dance around *Ballota africana* singing 'dis 'n lekker kruie' (O what a lovely herb).

Domestically, the dried square stems of black horehound were used as wicks for butterlamps or night lights, and the leaves burnt to drive off biting insects.

Most writers suggest that black horehound is no longer used, and that the white is better, but we find black horehound actually has a wider medicinal range.

Its champion is the early 20th-century English herbalist Richard Hool; contemporary American herbalist Matthew Wood deserves credit for highlighting Hool's well-argued passion for the plant.

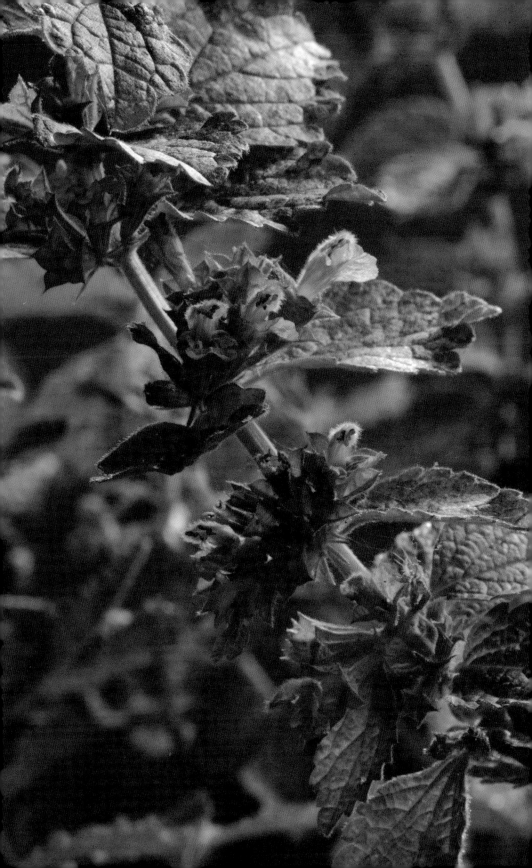

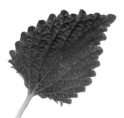

Black Horehound is one of the most efficacious remedies we have for the cure of biliousness, bilious colic, and sour belchings. In the above complaints it is as near a specific as any remedy well can be.
The relief it affords is both prompt and certain, for if only a leaf or a piece of the stem be chewed, and the juice swallowed, it will be found to act as if a current of electricity had passed into the stomach, allaying all the symptoms momentarily.
– Hool (1924)

... an excellent remedy for calming nausea and vomiting when the cause lies within the nervous system rather than in the stomach.
– Hoffmann (2003)

Hool gives a remarkable case where some postal workers requested his help for one of their co-workers who was down with the cholera – loss of control of the bowels, shivering, trembling, sweating, and weakness. ... He sent them off with ballota, telling them not to worry. By afternoon one of the men returned to say their co-worker was back at work, joking and laughing, as usual.
– Wood (2008)

Use black horehound for ...

One of the most useful actions of black horehound is in treating nausea, particularly arising from motion or travel sickness and from inner ear problems, where ginger might be considered. It is also a good match with ginger or mint.

The pungency and bitter flavour of black horehound indicate its benefits for digestion. It appears to increase the flow of bile and has a protective action on the liver. In southern Italy it was traditionally used in cases of malaria to treat the swollen spleen and liver that accompany the disease.

Black horehound's antispasmodic effect works well for menstrual cramps, and for normalising menstruation generally. It is helpful for treating irregular periods, and lack of menstruation as well as heavy periods [see box].

Like white horehound, black horehound is excellent for coughs. It is an expectorant, helping clear mucus out of the lungs, and as an antispasmodic is useful for dry, tickly coughs and asthma. In the past it was used to treat bronchitis as well as consumption (tuberculosis of the lungs).

We have found that it calms nervous over-activity, releasing muscle tension and anxiety. It can be helpful in cases of insomnia if the leaf tea is taken before bed.

Black horehound also has tonic properties, and makes a reputable remedy for tiredness and debility, low energy and general weakness, especially if accompanied by a loss of appetite. Hool also used it as a diuretic in treating oedema, and for internal gravel.

An ancient use, going back two thousand years to Dioscorides, was to bruise the leaves with salt to dress and heal dog bites (but this is not where 'hound' came from!). He also advocated mixing the leaves with honey for cleansing infected wounds and ulcers.

Black horehound as normaliser

In suppressed, and also in excessive, menstruation it is simply wonderful. It may seem contradictory to the ordinary reader to say that it may be prescribed in what are generally considered to be opposite conditions of the system; but when it is understood that in either case the disturbance of the physiological condition is simply due to a loss of equilibrium, and that the Black Horehound exerts such an influence as will restore the necessary equilibrium, it will be seen that it may be intelligently applicable to either case.

It should always be remembered that disease arises from obstruction, and that until this obstruction is removed and any injury to the part is repaired, there is always a disturbance of the equilibrium of the blood circulation and the nerve force.

– Richard Lawrence Hool, *Health from British Wild Herbs*, 1924 [1918]

Modern research

An Italian study (2010) found that extracts from three medicinal plants (*Ballota nigra*, *Castanea sativa* and *Sambucus ebulus*) were effective against MRSA. These anti-pathogenic plant extracts inhibited quorum sensing (QS) pathways, and may be a useful alternative to antibiotics in an age when increased bacterial resistance to antibiotics is a growing problem.

Animal and *in vitro* studies on species of *Ballota* have indicated its use to protect the liver, eg in a rat study (2008) *Ballota undulata* was found to lower blood glucose, increase insulin and reduce blood cholesterol levels.

A 2003 *in vitro* study compared the antimicrobial and antifungal effects of ethanol tinctures of 16 Turkish species of *Ballota*, finding they were 'good' antimicrobials and 'excellent' antifungals.

A 2014 study found *Ballota nigra* to be effective against the trypanosomatid protozoan parasite that causes Leishmaniasis.

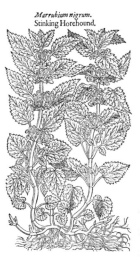

Marrubium nigrum.
Stinking Horehound.

Black horehound, woodcut in Gerard's *Herball* (1597)

Harvesting black horehound
The above-ground parts are used, especially the flowering tops, and can be gathered when flowering in summer and autumn. Use fresh to make tincture or dry for later use as tea.

Black horehound tincture
A simplified tincture method for fresh herbs can be followed: fill your chosen jar with **black horehound**, pressing it down to eliminate air pockets. Then add your **alcohol**, at a dilution of 20% of alcohol. We use diluted pure grain alcohol but commercial vodka is equally good. Half vodka and half water will give roughly the required dilution. Fill to the brim and push down any plant left sitting above the fluid level.

Leave your tincture bottle in a dark location for a month or so, at least until the plant content has been extracted. Pour the contents through a sieve into a clean bottle, stopper this and label. The flavour is slightly salty and sweet.

Dosage: a teaspoon three times a day. The taste is palatable, though still 'medicinal'.

Black horehound tea
Steep fresh or dried tops of flowering **black horehound** in **boiling water**, for 5 to 10 minutes, according to taste. It is pleasantly bitter.

Black horehound tincture
- muscle tension
- anxiety
- cramps
- low energy
- liver protective
- coughs
- bronchitis
- menstrual problems
- nausea

Black horehound tea
- stimulates digestion
- nausea
- coughs
- insomnia

Blackthorn *Prunus spinosa*

Rosaceae
Rose family

Description: A large shrub/small tree (to 4m, 14ft), suckering into dense thickets; simple oval leaves; black wood, bearing lateral shoots that develop into fearsome spines and from which delicate white blossoms with long golden stamens emerge in spring; these become small blue-black plums in autumn (the sloes).

Habitat: Woods, hedgerows, waysides, railway cuttings.

Distribution: Common in Britain, apart from Scottish Highlands. Widespread in Europe, western Asia, introduced to eastern North America, New Zealand.

Related species: Other European Prunus species, eg wild cherry (*Prunus avium*), cherry plum (*P. cerasifera*), bird cherry (*P. padus*). In North America, black cherry (*P. serotina*) and fire cherry (*P. pensylvanica*) are superficially similar.

Parts used: Flowers, bark, fruit (sloes).

Blackthorn's delicate white flowers are a reviving sight in spring, deserving their name 'lady of pearls'. A rose family astringent, its flowers are 'loosening' for intestinal pain whereas the fruit, or sloes, is 'binding' – a country remedy for diarrhoea, as well as gathered for the celebrated gin. Research is adding antioxidant and anti-tumour potential to its reputation.

The blackthorn is a wild ancestor of the cultivated plums, and is a relative of apricots, cherries, peaches and almonds. These were all classified by Linnaeus within the Prunus genus of the Rosaceae family.

Sloes, the fruit of blackthorn, have been dug up in Swiss lake dwellings dating from some 6,000 years ago. The famous mummy known as Ötzi, found in an Alpine glacier in 1991, and dated to 5,300 years ago, had stones from dried sloes near the corpse.

Unlike the cultivated Prunus species, blackthorn itself remains a wild, somewhat dangerous but valuable presence in hedgerows and woods.

Why use the emotive term 'dangerous'? The obvious answer is blackthorn's vicious thorns, which can be several inches long, and carry an old reputation of puncturing leather shoes or jerkins and causing wounds that never heal. A modern explanation is that when the thorn tip breaks off deep inside the skin it carries algal or fungal contamination. Infected blackthorn spines can introduce painful sinovitis and granuloma, often linked with fever.

Blackthorn wounds were so much part of everyday awareness that the translators of the King James Bible in 1611 were probably referring to blackthorn when talking of a 'thorn in the flesh', the 'messenger of Satan'.

Blackthorn was considered sinister in the 17th century for another reason, as the black wood staff was used by witches. A notorious example was the sorcerer Major Thomas Weir (1599–1670), who was burned at the stake in Edinburgh; his blackthorn rod, the agent of his magic, was thrown into the flames too.

Less dramatically, the dense wood of blackthorn made good teeth for hay rakes or walking sticks; in Ireland it was used as a club or shillelagh. Blackthorn burns well and slowly, and makes an impenetrable hedge.

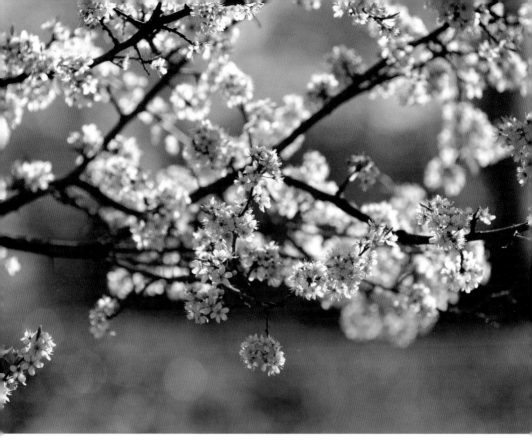

Use blackthorn for...

Blackthorn's early spring **flowers**, fresh and delicate, delight the eye with their lightness and prominent stamens; they were once called 'the lady of pearls'. They also have medicinal value for easing stomach and intestinal pain.

John Parkinson in 1640 wrote that drinking the distilled water of the flowers, preserved in white wine ('sacke') overnight, *is a most certain remedy tried and approoved, to ease all manner of gnawings in the stomacke, the sides, heart or bowells.*

Other former uses for blackthorn flowers include easing the pain and reducing the severity of cystitis and gravel, gout and dropsy (oedema). The effect is diuretic, laxative and 'loosening'.

Blackthorn **bark and roots** are highly astringent (as is the whole plant), and their tannins have been used to tan leather and make a black marker ink. Medicinally, they produce a strong decoction used to treat asthma and reduce fever. Blackthorn was among the country plants, alongside tormentil and blackberry, most often used against diarrhoea.

Blackthorn **leaves** are small and oval, much like ordinary tea, and indeed were once used as a tea adulterant. They make for a bitter drink or mouthwash and gargle for mouth ulcers. Used externally,

This spiny shrub ... might well be called 'the regulator of the stomach' since, by a happy scheme of nature, its flowers loosen the bowels and its fruits bind them.
– Palaiseul (1973)

At the end of October go gather up sloes, Have thou in readiness plenty of those, And keep them in bedstraw or still on the bough To stay both the flux of thyself and thy cow.

— anon, 19th century

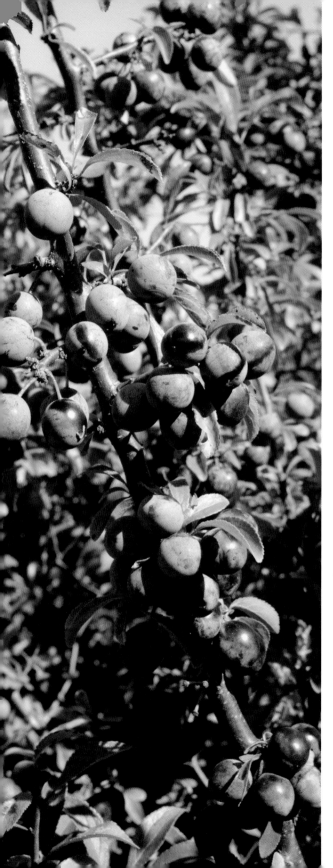

like any astringent, they will relieve skin inflammations.

Blackthorn **berries** or fruit are of course its sloes. Their taste was well described by Sir John Hill (1812): *very austere when unripe, but pleasant when mellow.* The old wives' tale of waiting for the first frost to sweeten the sloes is borne out by the chemical change induced by freezing conditions.

Freezing reduces the sloes' tannin levels and increases those of its sugars – whether you have collected your sloes and put them in the freezer or have left them on the bush. The astringency remains but the palatability improves, especially if the sloes are made into a syrup or wine.

Sloe wine was so tasty that, in the early 18th century, it was used *by fraudulent wine merchants in adulterating port wine. … It has been stated that there is more port wine (so called) drank in England alone, than is manufactured in Portugal.*

Julie's own experience bears out the tonic effects of the fruit. She was once recovering from appendicitis, and a German friend gave her a three times-decocted sloe syrup recipe. This settled her whole abdominal region.

Whereas the effect of blackthorn flowers is 'loosening' that of the sloes is 'binding', hence useful for treating cases of diarrhoea and dysentery and other bodily 'fluxes'. Sloes were also good against warts: a sloe was rubbed on the wart and then thrown over the shoulder. Sloes preserved in vinegar are a Western equivalent of the Japanese *umeboshi*, or dried, salted plums.

Modern research

Italian work in 2009 showed high antioxidant activity in fresh sloe juice, which acted as a cytoprotective.

Portuguese research (2014) using enriched phenolic extracts of wild fruits of sloes, strawberry tree and two species of rose displayed strong antioxidant and anti-tumour properties in each.

Isotonic drinks made separately from fruit of maqui, açaí and sloes, mixed with lemon juice, demonstrated higher antioxidant and biological effects than commercial isotonic drinks (2013).

A quick sloe syrup

Gather your **sloes** carefully in autumn, then freeze for a while. Transfer to a large jar; whatever your quantity, cover them with **vegetable glycerine**. Stopper the jar and place on a sunny windowsill. After about two months the liquid becomes a rich warm red. Drain off the depleted berries, put the syrup into a clean bottle, and label. Take a teaspoonful daily as a tonic.

Sloe spiced brandy

Don't be hung up on needing your sloes to be combined with gin: any alcohol is a good preservative.

A herbal friend tried this recently, tincturing **sloes**, **cardamom** and **fennel seeds** in **brandy**. The spices worked together beautifully, softening and mellowing the sloes' astringency; the bits of fruit left in the mixture tasted sweetish, rather like morello cherries.

A quick sloe syrup
- sore throats
- winter tonic
- disturbed digestion
- weak digestion

Sloe spiced brandy
- weak digestion
- dyspepsia
- lack of appetite
- sore throats
- winter tonic

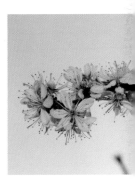

… the flowers of the blackthorn make the most harmless laxative and should be to the forefront of every family medicine chest. … So collect those blackthorn flowers, boil them for a minute, and drink a cupful of the infusion each day for three days. It acts very gently, without in any way upsetting your system; and yet it will purge you thoroughly. I recommend it also as a stomachic, depurative, and to fortify the stomach.
– Abbé Kneipp (1894)

Which thorn is it?

British people often say in late winter: Oh, the blackthorn is early this year. Usually they are wrong, because the first white-blossomed Prunus to appear in the hedgerow is cherry plum (*Prunus cerasifera*).

Cherry plum is taller than blackthorn (to 8m rather than 4m), lacks spines and is more open in habit; it has small dark red or yellow plums.

Blackthorn flowers generally appear (before the leaves) in massy drifts from early spring. Stems and branches are a dark wood, on which some side shoots form vicious spines 50cm (2in) or more long; blue-black fruits (sloes) follow.

The creamy white or pink flowers of hawthorn (*Crataegus monogyna*) appear later still when its leaves have already appeared, usually in May; hawthorn has shorter thorns than blackthorn, and red berries (haws). It is sometimes called May tree and whitethorn.

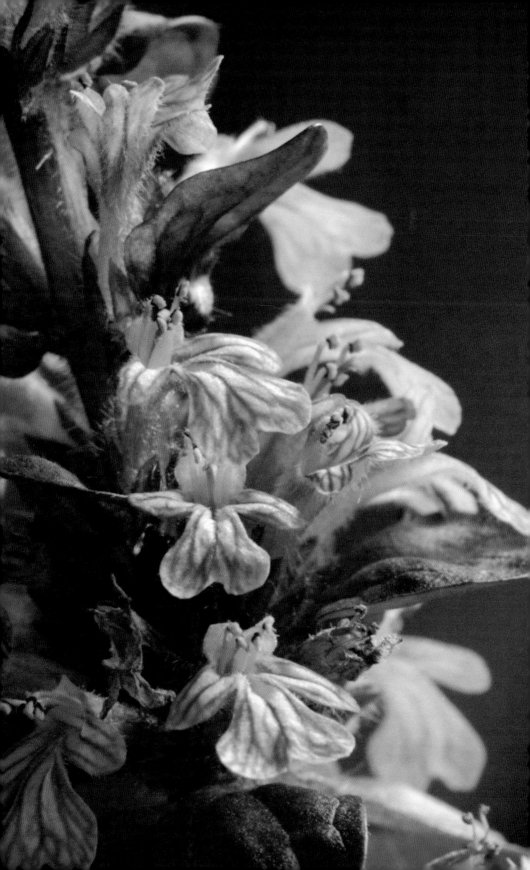

Bugle *Ajuga reptans*

Bugle was once one of the leading wound herbs, but this use is now all but forgotten. In our experience, bugle can be a useful treatment for aligning bones and dislocations, and it retains value as a mild analgesic and first aid standby.

**Lamiaceae
Deadnettle family**

Description: A creeping, colony-forming perennial with glossy dark green or purplish leaves, and blue flowers in whorls on spikes in spring and early summer.

Habitat: Found in woods and damp meadows.

Distribution: Common throughout the British Isles and across temperate Europe, north Africa and western Asia. Naturalised in the Americas and New Zealand.

Related species: There are over sixty species in the genus found around the world.

Parts used: Aerial parts.

Bugle is often grown in gardens as a ground cover for damp or shady places, and is available with purple and variegated leaves as well as the standard dark green. It spreads by extending stolons (runners) from the parent plant to form an attractive mat.

Gerard (1597) wrote that it was much planted in gardens in Elizabethan England, so it has been popular for a long time.

Bugle, sanicle and selfheal were reputed to keep the surgeon away, with many variations on the popular saying in herbal literature.

Because bugle is sometimes called bugleweed, it is often confused with the other plant of that name, *Lycopus virginicus* (see p96), but their uses are quite different.

Other common names include carpenter's weed and sicklewort, which indicate bugle's wound-healing properties in work situations, as does the old name of 'middle consound'. The consounds were wound-healing herbs, comfrey being the greater consound, and selfheal the lesser.

Use bugle for ...

In his English translation of the *Pharmacopoeia Londinensis* (1653) Nicholas Culpeper left no doubt about his admiration for bugle as a healing herb. He described it as excellent for falls and inward bruises for it dissolved congealed blood. It helped 'stoppings' (congestion) of the liver. It was of 'wonderful force' in curing

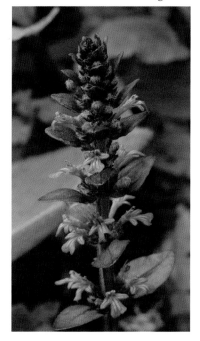

Bugle stands bravely on parade in the most cheerful and healthy colonies, in woods or in damp grass.
– Grigson (1958)

wounds and ulcers, and helping broken bones and dislocations. He added: *To conclude, let my Countrymen esteem it as a Jewel.*

Bugle had later champions, like the botanist Edward Baylis (1791), who devoted 13 pages of his herbal to its virtues, and particularly advocated it to treat the spitting of blood (as in incipient tuberculosis).

But after William Kemsey (1838) – who believed an ointment of bugle leaves and flowers was *good for all sorts of sores and old ulcers* – bugle seemed to slip out of official medical recognition. The gradual rise of antibiotics was one of the factors that led to the decline of herbal treatments for tuberculosis, and indeed wounds.

We would say the time is right to re-evaluate. It's good knowledge to have that bugle is a quietly effective first aid treatment for cuts, burns, bruising, sores and mouth ulcers or inflamed tonsils (quinsy). Scrunched-up bugle leaves on the affected part, either direct or via a wine decoction or poultice, are easily applied.

Pharmacological research shows bugle contains plentiful iridoid glycosides, including harpagide (as does the southern African herb devil's claw, *Harpagophytum procumbens*). Harpagide has a vasoconstricting effect on smooth muscle, which means both plants have blood-staunching properties.

Bugle is sometimes condemned as being only a mild analgesic. But let's rather say it is a safe one that acts gently to take the pain out of old wounds as well as fresh ones. We find it works well with a daisy ointment for bruises; with honey for sores and ulcers; and as a bugle distilled water for mouth issues.

Green's *Universal Herbal* of 1820 makes the interesting point that bugle is unlike most astringents when taken internally in that it does not produce costiveness (constipation), *but rather operates as gentle laxatives.*

Another role for bugle, we suggest, is as an alternative to the North American herb boneset (*Eupatorium perfoliatum*) for aligning bones, ligaments and tendons. This is less an innovation than recovering a traditional use (see quotes, left).

One experience of our own was that bugle tincture applied externally rapidly relieved a pinched nerve, while feeling more unctuous and tonic than boneset for the same purpose.

Modern research
Several traditional uses of closely related species of *Ajuga* have been confirmed in animal trials, and may well apply to *A. reptans*.

For example, *A. remota*, an anti-malarial herb in common use in East Africa, was shown (2011) to be effective in curing mice given doses of malaria; use of *Ajuga* in diabetes mellitus control was confirmed in diabetic rats treated by *A. iva*, a Mediterranean bugle species (2008a), with toxicity in the animals' livers, kidneys and pancreas much reduced.

Another species, *A. decumbens*, produced positive effects in Chinese research on osteoporosis and arthritis in mice (2008b), confirming traditional uses for human joint pain treatment.

These are laboratory findings rather than human clinical trials, of course, but how interesting to muse – and insist on appropriate research – whether *Ajuga reptans* shares potential with its cousins for treating malaria, diabetes, osteoporosis and arthritis.

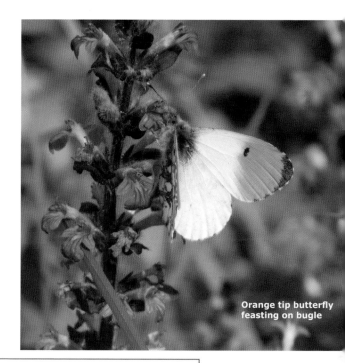

Orange tip butterfly feasting on bugle

Bugle tincture
Fill a jar with **bugle** flower spikes and leaves, then top up with 50% **vodka** or whisky and 50% **water**. Leave for a month or until the flowers have lost their colour, then strain, bottle and label.

Bugle elixir
Fill a jar with **bugle** flower spikes and leaves. Fill the jar ⅔ full with **vodka**, then top up with **vegetable glycerine**. Leave for a month or until the flowers have lost their colour, then strain, bottle and label.

Dosage: Take a teaspoonful three times daily.

Bugle ointment
Put **bugle** in a small saucepan with enough **extra virgin olive oil** to cover it. Simmer gently for about 20 minutes, then strain out the plant material. Measure the oil, and return it to the pan. Add 10g **beeswax** for every 100 ml of oil, and stir on low heat until melted. Pour into jars and allow to cool before putting the lids and labels on. Bugle combines well with daisy, yarrow and selfheal in an ointment.

Bugle tincture, externally
- back pain
- stiff necks
- joint pain
- injuries
- broken bones
- aching muscles

Bugle elixir
- hot liver
- gallbladder problems
- rapid heart beat
- anxiety
- persistent coughs

Bugle ointment
- cuts & grazes
- bruises
- blood blisters
- painful joints
- burns

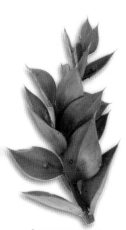

Butcher's broom *Ruscus aculeatus*

Asparagaceae
Asparagus family

Butcher's broom offers surprises in its family (it is an asparagus), form (its 'leaves' are modified stems) and palatability (it is a thorny plant with edible shoots). It had an engaging association with butchers which gave us its common name, and has enjoyed a surge of pharmacological interest for treating varicose veins and haemorrhoids, and potentially conditions of the lungs, liver and eyes.

Description: Multi-branched, hairless evergreen shrub, 1m tall (3ft); glossy, spiny, dark green 'leaves' or cladodes; tiny yellow-green flowers in centre of cladodes, then scarlet berries.

Habitat: Old woodland, hedgerows, cliffs, often at base of trees.

Distribution: Local, in lowland and southern Britain, most of Europe, western Asia.

Related species: Spineless butcher's broom (*R. hypoglossum*) is smaller, with more cladodes but fewer spines, and is a rare, introduced species.

Parts used: Root and cladodes.

A growing body of research is demonstrating that butcher's broom is a valuable medicine for venous disorders ... now a common remedy in Germany.
– Chevallier (2016)

Butcher's broom is a strange plant. Known in the past as knee holly because it is spiny and grows to about a metre tall, it superficially resembles but is not a holly. It is actually an asparagus, and an unusual one in that it is an evergreen bush.

The leaves of butcher's broom are modified stems (cladodes), its true leaves being vestigial. Its small yellow-green flower yields a cherry-like, non-edible red berry in the centre of the 'leaves'. These cladodes are leathery and tough, with a sharp terminal spine, yet the young shoots are reportedly edible, like a bitter form of asparagus.

Butcher's broom, as the name suggests, had an odd and old association with meat. It was reported by Parkinson (1640) that the Italian name for the plant was *Pongitopo*, and the German was *Muessdorn*, or mouse thorn. Italian and German butchers erected little 'hedges' of the 'leaves' around the meat to keep rodents away. The berries, which ripen in

autumn and stay on the bush over winter (or until birds eat them and spread the seeds), were once collected for Christmas décor and to garnish special cuts of meat. Florists have also used the berries. And indeed a switch or besom was once made from the stems to sweep the butcher's shop. Such uses are now long gone.

Use butcher's broom for ...
Butcher's broom was known as a medicinal plant to Dioscorides, the 1st-century AD herbal systematiser, and had a modest ongoing reputation as a diuretic and 'opening' herb for treating urinary, water retention, jaundice and stone or gravel issues.

In Devon, butcher's broom 'leaves' were used to beat chilblains, anticipating current uses of the plant for varicose vein treatment.

Herbalist Christine Herbert says: *My most common use is for congested menstrual problems – dysmenorrhoea/menorrhagia, as it is good for pelvic stagnation. It's also hormone-balancing, raising oestrogen and/or*

progesterone as needed. It's useful in
PMS, menopause, vaginal dryness.

Modern research
The isolation from butcher's broom of the steroidal saponin glycoside called ruscogenin has reinvigorated its medicinal status.

For example, 917 Mexicans with chronic venous disorder (CVD) were given 12 weeks of treatment with ruscogenin, with marked positive effects on their symptoms and quality of life (2009).

Ruscogenin and neoruscogenin have been shown to be effective in treating chronic venous insufficiency and chronic orthostatic hypotension (OH), the pooling of blood (2000).

The other major identified area is for relief of haemorrhoids, while more recent research suggests potential use for acute lung injury, pulmonary arterial hypertension, diabetic nephropathies and under-eye puffiness.

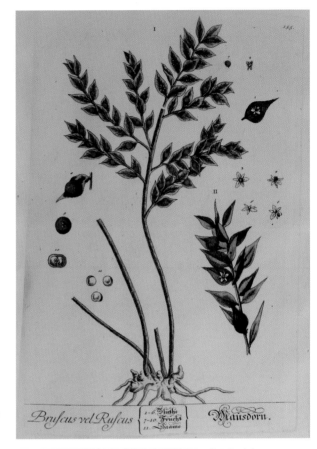

Butcher's broom, painted by Elizabeth Blackwell (1750), courtesy of the Wellcome Library

---

Butcher's broom infused oil
A tincure or tea are often made, but an alternative for external application to varicose veins and piles is an infused oil. Pick **butcher's broom cladodes** (and root if you must) and dry them in the shade. Put into a jar and pour on **extra virgin olive oil**. Stir well. Put the lid on and place the jar on a windowsill for 3 weeks or until the colour has transferred to the oil. Strain off the oil, bottle. Label.

Butcher's broom ointment
Mix 200ml of **butcher's broom infused oil** in a small saucepan and 20g **beeswax**. Warm on low heat until the wax melts, allow to cool slightly. Pour into jars and leave to set before putting lids on. Label.

Butcher's broom infused oil & ointment
• varicose veins
• chilblains
• piles

Caution: Do not eat the berries.

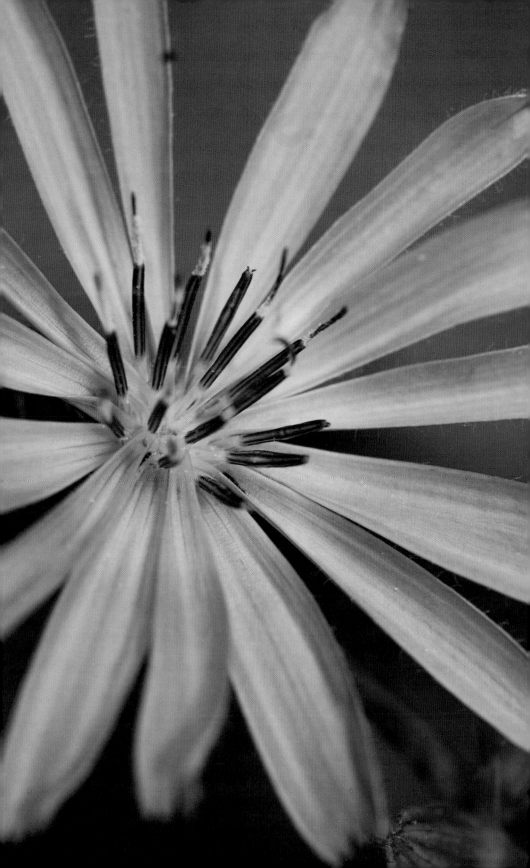

Chicory *Cichorium intybus*

Chicory is a familiar domestic presence as a coffee substitute and bitter salad ingredient, while the production of large-rooted varieties as a source of oligofructose is accelerating. These commercial emphases have overshadowed a well-established and significant herbal reputation.

Asteraceae
Daisy family

Description: A stiff-stalked perennial to 1.5m (4–5ft), with striking pale blue flowers scattered up the stem; leaves light green, lance-shaped at top, larger and lobed below; deep taproot.

Habitat: Along highways, waste and rough land, field margins, often near houses; likes lime soils.

Distribution: Widespread in lowlands of southern and eastern England, occasional elsewhere; native in Middle East and Mediterranean, now naturalised in North America, Asia, Australia.

Related species: Endive (*Cichorium endiva*) is a near-relative cultivated food crop, as is radicchio. Common blue sow thistle (*Cicerbita macrophylla*) is a scattered garden escape in Britain, but has lilac flowers, oval leaves and a white sap.

Parts used: Roots, leaves, flowers.

Chicory is an ancient herb of India, China, Iran, Egypt and the classical Mediterranean. It was a Passover 'bitter herb' of the Israelites and can still be found in Seder ceremonies today.

Pliny records both cultivated and wild chicory growing in ancient Rome, and recommended it for headaches and as a purgative. The influential medical writer Galen (c129–c210) wrote a *Treatise on Chicory*, drawing attention to its benefits for the liver, a use that has persisted to the present day. He recommended a syrup of chicory, rhubarb and oats for the liver.

Chicory is a morning kind of plant, which closes its long blue petals in the summer afternoons. Linnaeus included chicory in his floral clock at Uppsala, where it reliably kept the time; at his latitude in Sweden it opened at 5am and closed at 10am, while in Britain its hours are 6am to noon.

The great Arabic scientist Avicenna (980–1037) also wrote on chicory, and the species name *intybus* is an anglicisation of the Arabic name, *hendibeh*. Not wasting a good source-word, ancient plant-namers also transformed *hendibeh* into the related endive (*Cichorium endiva*).

The wild British and American chicory is the rough-stalked and blue-flowered species, once known as blue sailors or blue dandelion; another old English name was succory. This may have derived from the Latin *succurrere*, to run under, for chicory's depth of root.

Chicory's leaves are tender in spring, and can be foraged to be cooked or eaten fresh for their emerging bitterness; the flowers make a spectacular salad garnish. Endive hearts are blanched at an early stage to reduce their bitterness, while the related red radicchio now featuring in salads everywhere originated as a wild Italian chicory.

Chicory has become naturalised across most of North America, and is best known as a summertime highway weed. It is 'noxious' in some states, but loved by passers-by. It is *Wegwarten*, or watcher of the wayside, in Germany.

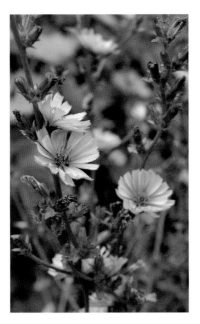

... the friend of the liver.
Galen (2nd century AD)

... a foremost remedy for the liver organ, whatever the condition.
– Holmes (2006)

Go early to bed, Drink Camp when you rise, You will be Healthy, Wealthy & Wise.
– early poster for Camp Coffee, c 1880s

The long taproot makes the familiar coffee substitute, often resorted to in times of blockade and coffee shortage, as in France during the Napoleonic Wars, the American South during the Civil War ('Creole' coffee) or in Britain in and after the Second World War.

'Camp' coffee, a mixture of 4% coffee, 28% chicory and sugar, first appeared in India in the 1870s as a stimulating drink for a Scottish regiment. This may have been the world's first instant coffee. It also makes excellent iced coffee.

Chicory root is cultivated commercially as a source of oligofructose, a high-fructose and low-calorie form of sugar. Some 100,000 tons is produced each year in the Netherlands, for use in weight-control formulae and as a substrate for probiotic gut bacteria, like acidophilus.

Use chicory for...
Medicinally, chicory has been valued in traditional herbalism around the world as a bitter tonic, with diuretic and decongestant effects similar to those of the closely related dandelion.

Chicory's effect is partly dose-dependent. American herbal energetics author Peter Holmes notes that *Smaller doses are restoring, while larger ones are more draining and detoxicant.*

Chicory root as a tea, coffee or syrup stimulates digestion and appetite. It is nourishing to the taste and to the blood, and helps relieve fatigue. It reduces congestion, especially in the liver, while promoting bile production – useful in jaundice treatments.

The root and also pressed chicory juice are cooling, with a detoxing and urine-promoting effect in higher doses, and help remove oedema. Chicory has been used to relieve gout and rheumatism. For children, chicory syrup was a mild and safe laxative.

Chicory leaf tea was taken to help reduce inflammations and fever, particularly fevers arising from congestive causes in the liver; in Traditional Chinese Medicine *ju ju* (chicory) corrects liver fire.

Older European traditions linked chicory with treating eye problems, including cataract. Fresh bruised leaves used to be applied on eye inflammations.

Interestingly, in TCM, the liver is strongly linked with the eye, so a 'liver herb' like chicory would be expected to be useful in both cases. In Indian tradition, juices of celery, carrot and chicory are drunk to support health of the optic nerve.

American scientist Jim Duke writes of research showing chicory reducing a rapid heartbeat but also being mildly heart-stimulating. It makes us wonder: could chicory be beneficially combined with hawthorn as a heart tonic?

Modern research
Immunotoxicity induced by ethanol was significantly restored or prevented in mice by *Cichorum intybus* treatment (2002). *C. intybus* hydroalcoholic extracts were effective (2012 research) to protect mice against experimental acute pancreatitis.

Ginger, chicory and their mixture were all found (2010) to be hepatoprotective against carbon tetrachloride intoxication in rats.

In a human study, trials with 47 people over 4 weeks showed (2015) that chicory root extract could delay or prevent the early onset of diabetes mellitus and improve bowel movement.

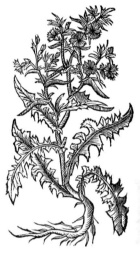

Wilde succory (chicory), woodcut in Parkinson, *Theatrum Botanicum* (1640)

Cardamom Camp coffee
Dig up your chicory root (this may be a tussle as it is a gnarly tap root), wash it and cut into small pieces (say 1cm or ¼ inch). It can be used fresh or roasted until it is brown, but we're going with drying it in a dehydrator (or the oven on low heat). Measure 4 tablespoons of this **dried chicory root**, 1 tablespoon **ground coffee beans**, 3 **cardamom pods** and 5 tablespoons **sugar** into 2 cups **water**. Boil and then simmer for 10 minutes. Allow to sit for 10 minutes, strain into a fresh saucepan. Simmer down to half volume – and at last you can bottle it. Keeps well in the fridge.

The result should be a thick syrup that is as good as any proprietary blend. The inulin starches have been transformed into caramelised sugars, while the cardamom tempers the bitterness.

Chicory skin toner
Pick a handful of **chicory leaves**. Mix sufficient solution of 2 parts **rosewater** and 1 part **cider vinegar** to cover the leaves. Run the mixture through a blender to make a dark green liquid. Strain into a fresh bottle. Use on the skin as a refreshing cosmetic and for minor skin blemishes.

Cardamom Camp coffee
- good for the liver
- stimulates digestion
- nourishing
- relieves fatigue

Chicory skin toner
- refreshing cosmetic
- minor skin blemishes

Cranesbill *Geranium* spp.

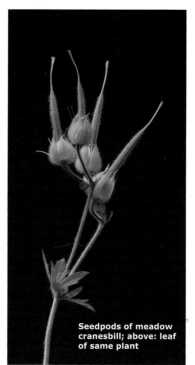

Geraniaceae
Geranium family

Description:
Cranesbills (*Geranium* spp.) and storksbills (*Erodium* spp.) are genuses within the Geranium family, with purple/pink/blue flowers and palmate (cranesbill) or pinnate leaves (storksbill); storksbills have longer 'beaks'.

Habitat: Grassland, woodland, rocks and cliffs, especially lime-rich areas.

Distribution: Cranesbill species are common across the British Isles, mainly in lowlands, storksbills less widespread; native to Mediterranean, Middle East, also North America, South Africa.

Related species: Herb robert (*Geranium robertianum*) is the most widespread British species [see p104], but meadow cranesbill (*G. pratense*), dovesfoot (*G. molle*), hedgerow (*G. pyrenaicum*), bloody (*G. sanguineum*) and cut-leaved cranesbill (*G. dissectum*) run it close. In eastern North America the main species is American or wild geranium (*G. maculatum*); a South African equivalent is *G. incanum* (*vrouebossie*).

Parts used: Rhizomes, leaves.

Two geranium species are most often used herbally: American cranesbill as a traditional astringent, and herb robert as a hedgerow medicine. Other wild geraniums have similar medicinal virtues and should not be forgotten.

The British native geraniums are known as cranesbills and storksbills. They are named for the comparison of the seedheads with the beaks of these once-familiar birds, and like the birds themselves may just be making a comeback.

Seedpods of meadow cranesbill; above: leaf of same plant

There is an almost universal confusion between the plants in the genus *Geranium* and those tender garden plants commonly called geraniums, which are *Pelargoniums*. They are both in the family Geraniaceae, and Linnaeus had included both groups of plants under the genus *Geranium*. They were separated into two genera by Charles L'Héritier in 1789. Pelargoniums are scented, and originated in warmer climes, particularly South Africa.

Back to real geraniums. Taking two leading twentieth-century herbals as a neglect baseline, there is some way still to go: Mrs Grieve (1931) covers *Geranium maculatum*, the American geranium, but no British species, not even herb robert (*G. robertianum*); Bartram (1995) has the American species and herb robert, but no others.

Two representative older herbals feature more species. Culpeper (1653) describes 'cranebil, the divers sorts of it' among the 'official' plants of the British pharmacopoeia; he relates the uses for dovesfoot cranesbill (now *G. molle*) and adds, *I suppose*

Colony of bloody cranesbill, County Clare, June

these are the general vertues of them all. Salmon (1707) itemises four garden and six wild cranesbills, saying confidently: *The Qualities, Specification, Preparations, Virtues and Uses, of all the Cranes-bills, being one and the same…*

Our forefathers evidently valued many more geranium species for their medicine, and thought their properties were broadly similar. We think that the over 400 wild geranium species worldwide (including in Britain at least 26 cranesbills and 12 storksbills) deserve some recognition.

Use cranesbills for…
As in herb robert (p104), the phytochemical signature of cranesbills is their astringency – American geranium roots have some 10–20% tannin content.

The effect of taking a cranesbill root or leaf tea, tincture or other formulation is primarily to control bodily discharges ('fluxes'), such as chronic diarrhoea, excessive menstruation and other forms of bleeding, flowing mucus and hyperacidity in the stomach (including peptic ulcers).

American herbalist Jim Mcdonald summarises his local Midwest geranium as 'a gastrointestinal astringent', which is especially good for 'tightening damp wounds in the intestines'. British botanical writer Deni Bown suggests combining American geranium with avens (*Geum*

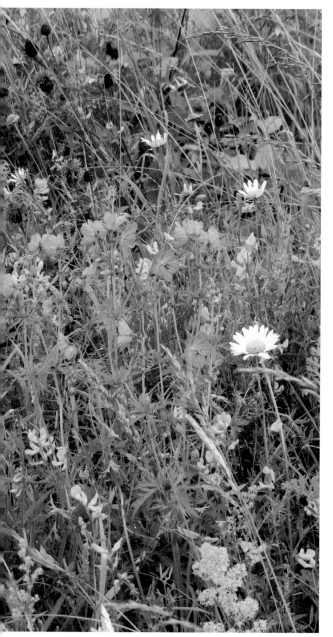

urbanum) to treat bleeding in the digestive tract and internal ulcers.

American herbalist Peter Holmes summarises American geranium (and we would suggest other species) as being 'mucostatic and hemostatic', adding piles, vaginitis and mouth ulcers as areas for its action. The late Michael Moore found crushed or powdered American geranium root as a paste helps draining of pus in wounds, gum disease or external sores.

In South Africa *Geranium incanum* is 'vrouebossie' (woman's bush), because a tea made of the leaves is a folk remedy for heavy menstruation and diarrhoea, mirroring traditional uses in Europe and among Native Americans in North America.

Another South African native relative, *Pelargonium graveolens*, or rose geranium, is a leading commercial essential oil used medicinally for similar purposes.

Mcdonald notes that American geranium roots are easily pulled up for medicine-making, and can be moderated by cooking them in milk or with cinnamon. Picking herb robert, too, can hardly be easier as it has convenient stem clusters. What are we waiting for?

Modern research
Russian work (2007) found that polyphenols in geranium and rose family species are antibacterial via antioxidant action.

Mexican research (2015) on *G. schiedeanum*, a local species of geranium, displayed hepatoprotective (liver-protecting) effects in rats by reduction of ethanol-induced toxicity.

Similarly, *Geranium macrorrhizum*, widely used in Balkan folk medicine, showed hepatoprotective potential as an antimicrobial, in addition to its astringent, wound-healing properties (2012).

Cranesbill ointment

Pick whichever **cranesbill** is abundant where you are. The roots will be stronger, but the above-ground parts work perfectly well.

Place in a small saucepan with enough **extra virgin olive oil** to cover the plant material. Heat gently for about half an hour or until the plant material is losing its colour and starting to become brittle. Strain the oil through a sieve into a measuring jug.

Place in a clean pan with 10g **beeswax** or 5g **candelilla wax** per 100ml of oil, and stir over low heat until the wax has all melted. Pour into jars, allowing to solidify before putting the lids on and labelling.

Herb robert and yarrow combine well with cranesbill in this ointment, as do any of the rose family astringents such as rose, agrimony, silverweed, cinquefoil and tormentil.

Use for haemorrhoids (piles), cuts and grazes.

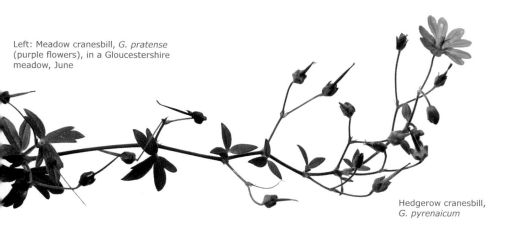

Left: Meadow cranesbill, *G. pratense* (purple flowers), in a Gloucestershire meadow, June

Hedgerow cranesbill, *G. pyrenaicum*

Creeping jenny *Lysimachia nummularia*
& Yellow loosestrife *Lysimachia vulgaris, L. punctata*

**Primulaceae
Primrose family**

Description: Creeping jenny is just a few inches high, but its creeping prostrate stems can be 50cm (18in) long; yellow cupped flowers and rounded opposite leaves; yellow loosestrife (*L. vulgaris*) is a tall, erect plant (to 150cm, 5ft), with pyramidal clusters of yellow flowers, lance-shaped narrow leaves. Dotted loosestrife (*L. punctata*) is very similar, but flowers have an orange centre and it prefers drier ground.

Habitat: Creeping jenny is found in damp, shady woods and wetter grassland; yellow loosestrife (*L. vulgaris*) in marshes, by streams and rivers; (*L. punctata*) damp places, verges, woodland margins.

Distribution: European natives, fairly common in central and southern England, and in Wales; introduced widely in US.

Related species: Yellow pimpernel (*Lysimachia nemorum*) is a widespread creeping yellow *Lysimachia*. 'Gold money herb', *jin qian cao* (*L. christinae*) is a medicinal Chinese relative.

Parts used: Above-ground parts.

Creeping jenny and yellow loosestrife are related members of the Primula family, one spreading laterally and other vertically to make imposing and attractive colonies. They share similar effectiveness in treating wounds and bleeding, 'fluxes' of various kinds and kidney and gall stones.

These two attractive yellow plants in the Lysimachia genus of the Primrose family are considered together. The first spreads out horizontally and the second forms strong vertical lines, but both have visually striking yellow and green contrasts, and share similar medicinal uses.

Neither is related to purple loosestrife, now classified in the Lythrum genus. The separate chapter on purple loosestrife (p139) looks at the reclassification and the Latin and popular names for the two loosestrifes.

As to 'loosestrife' itself, from the reputed use of the foliage to deter biting insects and hence calm restive oxen, John Parkinson (1640) comments trenchantly: *which how true I leave to them shall try, and finde it so.*

One other common name for creeping jenny deserves mention – 'moneywort'. Mrs Grieve suggests this arises from the roundish shape

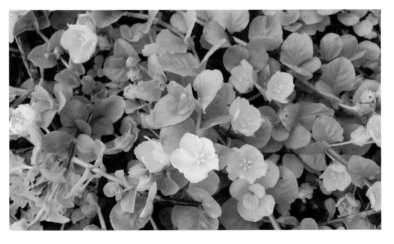

of the leaves, as they ascend the stem in pairs, resembling rows of pence. The money link is traced to William Turner (1548), the first to name the plant 'Herbe 2 Pence' and 'Two pennigrasse' (from the German *Pfennigkraut*), and confer the Latin form *nummaria* (coin).

Mrs Grieve (1931) speculates that another popular name, 'string of sovereigns', refers to the plant's golden flowers. 'Meadow runagates' and 'wandering sailor', other old vernacular names, reflect creeping jenny's spreading habit.

Use creeping jenny & yellow loosestrife for...
Those who think of creeping jenny as only a garden plant might be surprised at its medieval herbal reputation. It was known in France as a *herbe aux cent maux*, a plant for a hundred ills, in fact a panacea. It was a medicinal standby for many of the non-life-threatening but still significant things that happen. And of course it is still good for these same niggling interruptions to daily life, even if it has gone out of fashion itself.

Creeping jenny has been used since classical times, which makes its herbal history older than that of yellow loosestrife. It has generally been seen as more effective in the same healing areas. Culpeper (1653) summarises these: *Money-wort or Herb Two-pence; cold dry, binding,*

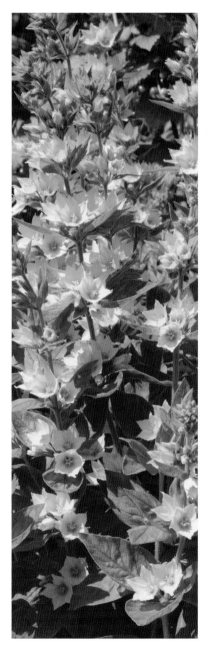

[Creeping jenny is] *singular good for to stay all fluxes of blood in man or woman, whether they be laskes* [diarrhoea], *bloody fluxes* [dysentery], *the flowing of womens monethly courses, or bleedings inwardly or outwardly, also the weaknesse of the stomacke, that is given to casting* [vomiting].
– Parkinson (1640)

[Yellow loosestrife is] *a wild plant not uncommon in our watery places, but for its beauty, very worthy a place in our gardens. If it were brought from America, it would be called one of the most elegant plants in the world.*
– Hill (1812)

Creeping jenny (far left); dotted loosestrife *L. punctata* (left), the yellow loosestrife most commonly grown in gardens

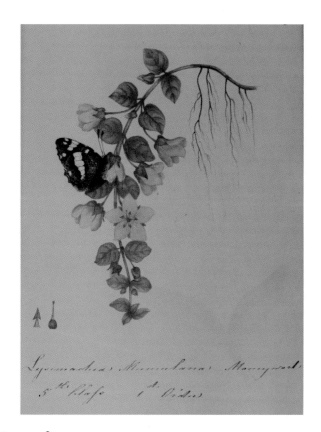

helps Fluxes, stops the Terms, helps ulcers in the lunges; outwardly it is a special herb for wounds.

We would now say both plants are astringent, vulnerary, diuretic and antiscorbutic.

The astringency or binding property comes into play to help stop 'fluxes' of all kinds, whether upset stomach, diarrhoea or dysentery ('bloody flux').

As vulneraries, both plants healed wounds by stopping bleeding, whether old or new wounds, flowing or not, ranging from nose bleeds to piles or excess menstruation and 'whites' (leucorrhoea).

As diuretics, both plants increase urine flow, helping reduce the pain of kidney or gallstones and in some cases expel them.

Both were seen as useful against scurvy (as antiscorbutics), though their saponins, especially in yellow loosestrife, made the medicine taste soapy without added honey.

Another area of action for both plants includes the mouth, as a mouthwash for mouth ulcers, bleeding gums and quinsy (sore throat), and the lungs.

Various means have been used to take the herbs, including sipping the juice, a decoction in water or wine, the powder dissolved in water, and using the juice as a

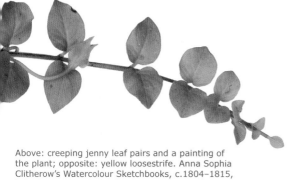

Above: creeping jenny leaf pairs and a painting of the plant; opposite: yellow loosestrife. Anna Sophia Clitherow's Watercolour Sketchbooks, c.1804–1815, John Innes Historical Collections, courtesy of the John Innes Foundation

skin wash or cold compress. Fresh leaves can be applied to wounds direct or an ointment made.

L. christinae, jin qian cao, or 'gold money herb', is a related Chinese plant used to promote urination, reduce jaundice and help to expel kidney stone and gallstones. The leading Western book on Traditional Chinese Medicine describes it as *a very important herb for treating stones in both the urinary and biliary systems.*

Modern research

An aqueous extract of *Lysimachia christinae* was found to have potent hyperuricemic effects on mice (2002), ie to lower very high levels of uric acid in the blood.

At least four new saponins have been identified in Lysimachia species since 2006. In 2013 a new glycosylated triterpene 1 (named nummularoside) was isolated from the roots of *Lysimachia nummularia*. This saponin had significant activity against prostate cancer cells and glioblastoma (a form of brain cancer), while not affecting normal cells.

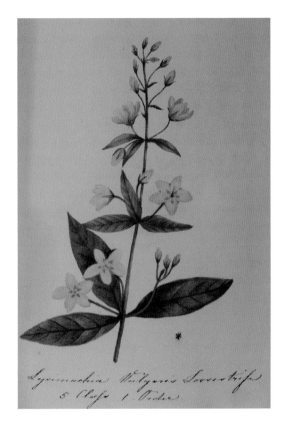

Lysimachia Vulgaris Loosestrife 5 Class 1 Order.

Twopenny tea

A healing tea is made from fresh or dried leaves and flowers of either plant. Scrunch up a handful of herb, put into a teapot, add boiling water and brew for 5 minutes. The leaves have some astringency and 'soapiness', so the taste will usually benefit from addition of honey or sugar. The effect should be soothing (demulcent) and settle upset stomachs or diarrhoea.

The cooled tea can be used as a gargle for sore throats or inflamed gums, and as a compress to place on surface wounds or skin sores. Alternatively, as with plantain, the bruised leaves themselves can be applied to the affected part.

Twopenny tea
- upset stomach
- diarrhoea
- sore throat
- minor wounds

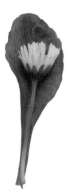

Daisy *Bellis perennis*

Daisies have long been enjoyed by poets and children, but gardeners are not so enthusiastic about the migration of these small plants from meadow to lawn. Medicinally, daisies have a somewhat neglected reputation for treating wounds, bruises and coughs, and as pain relievers. Recent clinical trials, however, offer exciting possibilities for using daisies in anti-oxidant, anti-microbial and anti-tumoural contexts.

Asteraceae
Daisy family

Description: A small perennial with rosettes of leaves hugging the ground. Flowers usually white, sometimes with red or pink on backs of petals. Petals close up at night and in cloudy weather.

Habitat: Short grass, including lawns.

Distribution: Native and common in the British Isles, Europe and western Asia. Introduced to North America.

Related species: There are 10 species in the genus *Bellis*.

Parts used: Leaves and flowers.

The daisy is universally known in temperate climes, but is sometimes specified as the English, common or lawn daisy. It is a close relative of the ox-eye daisy (see p124), and has similar medicinal uses.

Anne Pratt, the Victorian botanical writer and illustrator, explains the plant's popularity. She wrote in 1866: *How thoroughly the little wild flower is loved is told by the fact that never a poet, either of old or modern times, who has written of Nature, has forgotten to give it a line of praise.*

There's something in this. Daisy was the *dæges eage* (day's eye) to the Anglo-Saxons, and Chaucer in 1386 set the standard of affection – and confirmed daisy's status as a meadow plant: *That, of al the floures in the mede, / Thanne love I most thise floures white and rede, / Swiche as men call daysyes in our town.*

Other poets followed. Milton wrote in 1645 of *Meadows trim with daisies pied.* Shelley in 1822 called daisies *those pearled Arcturi of the earth / The constellated flower that*

never sets, while in 1821 John Clare had *daisies' silver studs / Like sheets of snow on every pasture spread.*

Mrs Pratt also had a thought about why it was so easy to love the common daisy: *Perhaps there is scarcely another* [flower] *which has power to awaken so fully the memories of early life. ... It is truly the bairnwort, the child's flower.*

The daisy is the right size for a child, and making daisy chains remains a familiar part of many children's experience. There's a story that Augustine, first archbishop of Canterbury (died AD 604), saw children outside the town busy threading daisies, and took the opportunity to preach the new religion, explaining that the golden centre of the flower was God the Father and the rays were good Christian souls.

Augustine was subtly offering a counter-ideology, a conversion narrative. The old belief was that daisies needed to be joined because evil spirits will not pass

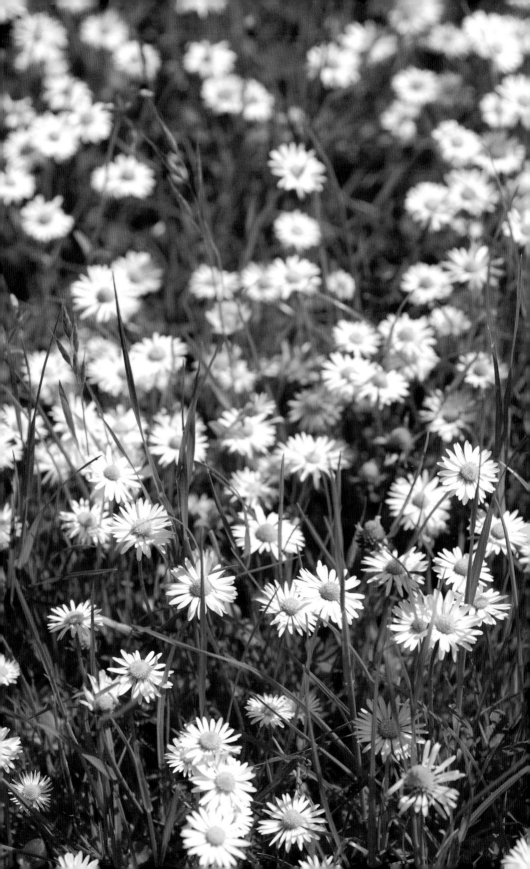

through a circle; hence daisy garlands, crowns, necklaces, bracelets and rings. This meant the daisies could be worn, and thereby prevent children of both sexes from being stolen by Little Folk, especially at May Day, when the faery kingdom is closest to us.

Some may dismiss this as 'paganism', but the passing down of daisy-chain skills from older to younger children is still with us. And so is the 'divination', if you will, of pulling off white daisy florets to the chant of 'he/she loves me, he/she loves me not'.

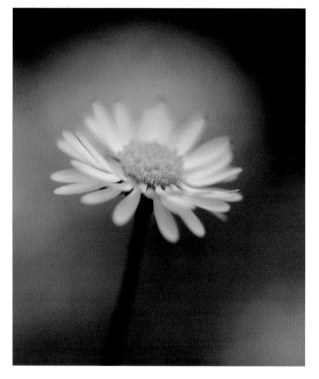

In the adult world, daisy is a plant that needs the grass around it to be short, hence its appearance in grazed meadows and of course in lawns. Despite concerted uprooting, poisoning and beheading, it always returns, shining brightly, through most of the year, available to us as a forgotten but readily available healing plant.

It seems ironic that people try to kill this wild tiny aster or chrysanthemum in the lawn while working hard to keep its garden cousins flowering in the borders. But we have noticed that daisy seems to be spreading out from the garden and college lawn and back into the meadow. A decade ago we spotted wild daisies in Dartmoor and remarked how unusual that was. Nowadays we see them far more widely, and expect you do too.

Use daisy for ...
As a modern woman of a hundred and fifty years ago, Mrs Pratt says of the older medicinal uses of the plant – she mentions for oils, ointments and internal medicines – *that the men of our days have done wisely in rejecting them*. We could not disagree more.

Back in Roman times, army surgeons organised the collection of daisies by slaves to extract the juice. Bandages soaked in this juice treated sword and spear wounds. This means the plant could have links with the Latin name *bellum*, war, though most still prefer the alternative of *bellis* for beautiful.

No matter, daisy maintained a strong reputation as a wound-healing herb, often used as an ointment or salve. Parkinson wrote (1640) *that an ointment made thereof doth wonderfully helpe all wounds, that have inflammations about them, or by reason of moist humours having accesse unto them, are kept long from healing.*

Parkinson here draws our attention to daisy's cooling and drying nature, and this applies too for its renown as 'bruisewort' when used for easing the heat and pain of bruises, ulcers, skin swellings and burns. We made a daisy and mugwort ointment for an inflamed cyst on Matthew's neck, with excellent results.

Daisy is a traditional expectorant, which taken as an infusion relaxes spasms presenting as coughs and catarrh or colic. It is also a mild diuretic, which helps relieve the pain of gout and arthritis.

Daisy leaves can be used direct on the skin as a poultice for tired muscles, or added to a hot bath for generic pain relief. Gerard advocated daisies *stamped* [pressed] *with new butter unsalted*

... a wound herbe of good respect, often used and seldome left out in those drinkes or salves that are for wounds, either inward or outward.
– Parkinson (1640)

Below: Daisy therapy with Kaz

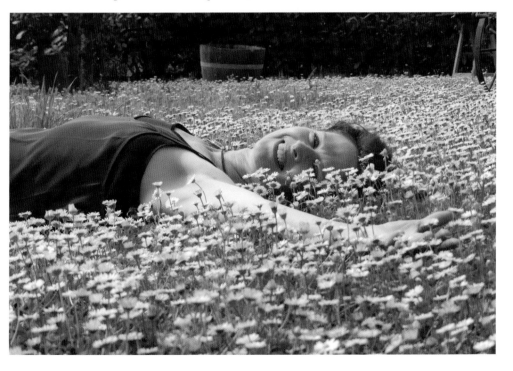

for painful joints and gout, while Parkinson preferred a tea from daisies, dwarf elder and agrimony.

A time-honoured use of daisy was to treat eye inflammations. John Wesley (1765) has a recipe (see left) that claims efficacy even *tho' the Sight were almost gone.*

Daisy is a close relative of arnica (*Arnica montana*), and is sometimes called 'poor man's arnica' as a pain reliever. Irish-based herbalists Nikki Darrell and Chris Gambatese find daisy to be the more effective, as do we. It has the added benefit of being free and local, and without toxicity.

Former internal uses for daisy in treating inflamed liver and bruising in pregnancy have dropped away, and indeed modern advice is against taking daisy internally in pregnancy.

Daisy leaves in salads add a succulent presence and a soapy or sour tang, with the white florets a bright final garnish. Herbalist Anne McIntyre likes a daisy soup, using the flowers and leaves, with added stock and ginger.

Modern research
Remarkable strides are being taken in clinical trials using daisy. Some examples:

- Daisy ointment healed wounds without scarring in 12 rats, the first scientific verification of the plant's traditional wound-healing activity (2012).
- Flavonoids isolated from daisy flowers showed strong *in vitro* antioxidant potential (2013).
- Antimicrobial activity of daisy essential oils was demonstrated (1997).
- Anti-tumour activity from saponins in daisy was shown for the first time (2014).
- Seven triterpine saponins were newly isolated from daisy flowers (2016). One of them, perennisaponin O, *exhibited anti-proliferative activities against human digestive tract carcinoma.*
- Homeopathic *Arnica montana* and *Bellis perennis* may reduce postpartum blood loss (2005).

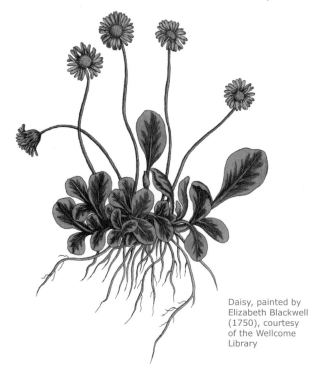

Daisy, painted by Elizabeth Blackwell (1750), courtesy of the Wellcome Library

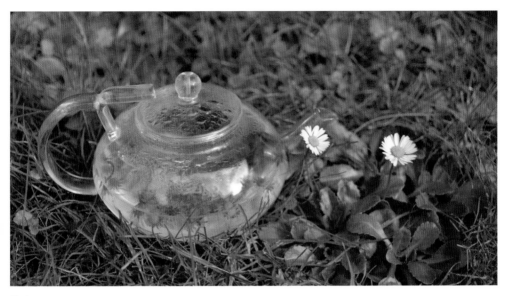

Daisy tea

While daisies can be found in flower for much of the year, we usually pick them in the spring when they are abundant, and dry them for use as a tea. Use a heaped teaspoonful of dried **daisy flowers** per mug of **boiling water**. Cover and let stand for about 10 minutes, then strain and drink. We find daisy tea has similar properties to the more familiar chamomile.

Combine with ground elder for gout and arthritis.

A daisy ointment

Make an infused oil of daisies by filling a jam jar with fresh or dried **daisies**. Pour on enough **extra virgin olive oil** to cover the flowers; press down to remove air pockets. If you have used fresh daisies, cover the jar with a cloth held on by a rubber band – this allows any moisture to escape. With dried daisies you can just use a normal jar lid.

Leave on a sunny windowsill to infuse for about a month. Then strain out the flowers, add 10g **beeswax** for every 100ml of oil, and heat gently until the beeswax has melted. Check for setting by putting a drop on a cold saucer. If too soft, add a little more beeswax. When ready, pour into clean jars and allow to cool before putting the lids on. Label.

Mugwort, plantain and yarrow also work well with daisy.

Daisy tea
- relaxing
- coughs
- painful joints
- gout

Daisy ointment
- bruising
- cuts
- grazes
- sore muscles

Caution
Avoid taking daisy internally in pregnancy

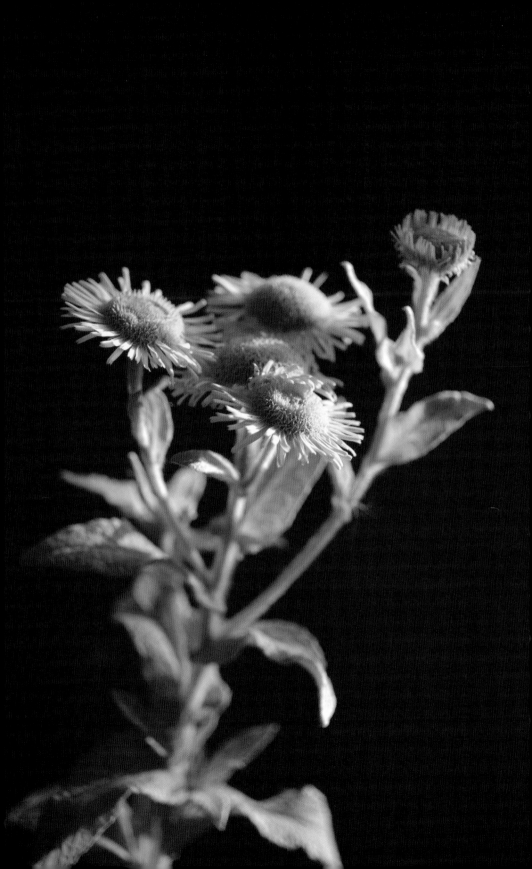

Fleabane *Pulicaria dysenterica*

Herbal names sometimes tell most of the story of a particular plant's effectiveness. Fleabane is a good example, with names reflecting traditional roles as an insecticide or repellant and for treating dysentery. It shares other medicinal actions with related members of the Aster family that should widen its use.

Fleabane is a somewhat elusive name, as it could refer to species in any of five genera within the huge family of Asters (or daisies, once called the Compositae).

These five genera are the *Inula* (notably elecampane and ploughman's spikenard); the *Dittrachia* (woody and stinking fleabane); the *Pulicaria* (common and the rare small fleabane); the *Erigeron* (blue and Mexican fleabane); and the *Conyza* (Canadian fleabane).

Our focus here is on *Pulicaria dysenterica*. The names tell it like it is: the common fleabane really does kill fleas (*Pulex* is the Latin for flea), and it has been used to tackle epidemics of dysentery.

It was Linnaeus who conferred the species name 'dysenterica', in the mid-18th century, after hearing from General Keit, a Russian army commander, that the plant had cured his soldiers of dysentery on a campaign against the Persians.

Plant names are often changed but specific medicinal qualities can persist through time and space, and remain valid today, even if the benefits are generally forgotten.

It should be no surprise that a fleabane relative (probably an *Inula*, elecampane) in Pharaonic Egypt was ground up with charcoal and the dust spread over the house to expel fleas.

Egyptian homes were plagued by rats, mice and fleas, and while cats were good against rodents, it took natron (sodium) water or fleabane to tackle fleas.

Fleas are always a corollary of civilisation, for where man goes so do they. Beds, whether of feathers for a king or straw for a peasant, attract biting creatures of various kinds, especially in the summer.

And fleas require a human response, although it was not known until relatively recent times that fleas carried bubonic plague bacteria, and nor was the link understood between mosquitoes and ague or malaria. But people were all too aware that fleas and midges were pests, and

Asteraceae
Daisy family

Description: Medium, untidy perennial (to about 50cm, 20in), with downy, grey-green foliage and bright yellow flowers, with flat tops and thin ray florets, above wrinkled erect leaves.

Habitat: Damp, often rough grassland, wayside ditches.

Distribution: Native to Europe and Western Asia; in Britain, southwards from Yorkshire and Lancashire (the obverse of goldenrod, which flourishes north of this area).

Related species: Many, including elecampane (*Inula helenium*), goldenrod (*Solidago virgaurea*), Canadian horseweed (*Conyza canadensis*), blue fleabane (*Erigeron acer*).

Parts used: Above-ground parts, juice, essential oil.

... though in England it [common fleabane] has never had much reputation as a curative agent it has ranked high in the estimation of herbalists abroad.
– Grieve (1931)

apothecaries like John Parkinson, writing in 1640, prescribed fleabane – for, *being burnt or laid in Chambers* [bedrooms], *it will kill Gnats, Fleas, or Serpents, as Dioscorides saith.*

The referencing of classical authority was typical of Parkinson, and he added that fleabane leaves were to be used for *bytings or hurts of all venemous creatures, as also for pushes* [pimples] *and small swellings, and for wounds.*

At that time fleabane was dried and hung in bunches in houses, or burnt in the hearth. The smell was camphorous and rather unpleasant, but as long as it killed the pests (insecticide) or deterred them (repellent) it was tolerated.

This is domestic medicine, but a close Aster relative of fleabane is the commercial-scale *Tanacetum cinerarifolium*. Once grown in the Balkans and now in Kenya, the flowerheads of this plant yield the leading non-synthetic and organic insecticide, pyrethrum.

Use fleabane for ...
Are there other uses for fleabane, apart from helping with fleas and dysentery? Parkinson hinted above at a role as a wound herb, appropriate for an astringent, and relevant for many

medicinal plants among the wider Aster family.

Aster relatives, like the Canadian fleabane (*Erigeron canadensis*), are known and used for staunching blood flow topically, including for irregular menstrual bleeding and local haemorrhaging. The essential oil of this plant is often recommended in such situations, as antimicrobial and antibacterial.

The same is true for common fleabane, which ties back to its effectiveness against fleas and the pathogens they carry, no less than in treatment of dysentery.

Parkinson again: his list of virtues for fleabane included treating skin eruptions, as we have seen, and he said an extract of its leaves and flowers, boiled in wine, would help disturbed urine flow and counteract jaundice and griping pains.

In terms of method, he said the plant's juice could be swallowed and a tea or tincture made of the above-ground parts. A bath that included a quantity of the tea would be beneficial, while the distilled oil of the plant could be anointed (rubbed on the forehead) for 'fits of agues' (malarial fevers) and cold trembling.

Parkinson also cautioned that fleabane was a stimulant for the 'mother' (womb), and could cause spontaneous abortion. This warning should still be heeded.

The green leaves [of fleabane] *made into a pultice, by beating in a Mortar, & applied to any simple green Wound, or Cut, being first well washed or cleansed, heals it in a very short space of time ...*
– Salmon (1710)

Fleabane, painting by Rudolf Koch and Fritz Kredel (1929), John Innes Historical Collections, courtsey of the John Innes Foundation

Modern research

Ethnobotanical research seems to support Parkinson's findings. An allied species, *Pulicaria crispa*, is known in contemporary Pakistan as 'bui', and is used in syrup form to treat jaundice, ulcers, wounds and itchy skin (2012).

Research (1992) in Baluchistan found another species, *P. glaucescens* ('kulmeer'), being used in post-parturition care for women. It was boiled with other herbs, and 'gur' (raw sugarcane) added; the paste was rolled out and inserted into the vagina.

Pharmacological research has also confirmed aspects of the traditional profile. Iranian studies (2014a) on fleabane essential oil showed that it inhibited all micro-organisms tested, except for salmonella and shigella, and was partly effective against *E. coli*.

Saudi Arabian *in vivo* research (2014b) found *P. glutinosa*, another close fleabane relative, to be neuroprotective in zebra fish; the authors suggested fleabane be studied relative to human degenerative diseases, eg Parkinson's and Alzheimer's.

Caution
Avoid fleabane in pregnancy as it may stimulate the uterus.

Flea repellant bag

Fresh or dried **fleabane** can be put in a pillowcase or small **cloth bag** to deter fleas from biting in bed. Simply place the bag in the bed or under a pillow. We have found this practice very effective.

A small bag of fleabane can also be tucked into clothing or carried in a pocket to repel fleas during the day.

Fleabane tea

Pick a 3-inch sprig of fresh **fleabane** per mug of **boiling water**, and steep for 5 or 10 minutes before drinking.

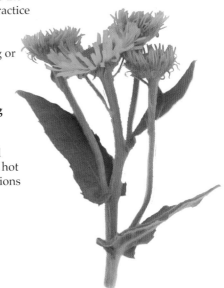

This tea has surpisingly little flavour but is smooth and soothing. A larger quantity of the tea can be added to a hot bath to ease itching from a biting insect or minor irritations of the skin.

Fleabane tea
- cystitis
- infections
- dry tickly coughs
- griping pains

Forget-me-not *Myosotis arvensis*

German legends, a poet with a footnote and a steamy scene from DH Lawrence: forget-me-not is irresistible to writers! It may sound dull after all this that the plant's predominant medicinal use is a cough syrup and as a flower essence, but clinical research is now suggesting other prospects.

Boraginaceae
Borage family

Description: Annual/perennial, typically less than 50cm (20in) tall; thin hairy stems; small, terminal flowers, of striking pale blue with yellow 'eye'; daisy-like spatulate leaves; prolific in spring and summer.

Habitat: Generally fields, woods, waysides, gardens.

Distribution: Native in Eurasia and New Zealand; naturalised in US, apart from south and southwest.

Related species: Water forget-me-not (*Myosotis scorpioides*, syn. *M. palustris*) retains the old allusion to scorpions in its name, and is found at pond edges and in damp fields; wood forget-me-not (*M. sylvatica*) prefers drier rock and woodland habitats; *M. arvensis* var. *sylvestris* is the larger-flowered garden variety. Half a dozen more species are known in Britain, and about a hundred worldwide.

Parts used: Flowering tops, stems and leaves.

There is an old German legend in which God was naming all the flowers. One, a little blue flower, was overlooked. It called out, 'Forget-me-not', and God said that as all the names had gone, these very words were to be its name.

There was confusion about the plant for over 1500 years after Dioscorides (1st century AD) used the common name of 'mouse-ear' (*myosotis*), which also applied to

a type of hawkweed. John Gerard (1597) named three *Myosotis* species, but there was as yet no agreed common name.

It needed the poet Samuel Taylor Coleridge to give the plant the name we know it by today. Coleridge was travelling in Germany in the early years of the 19th century. He knew the medieval German legend of a love-struck knight, who was

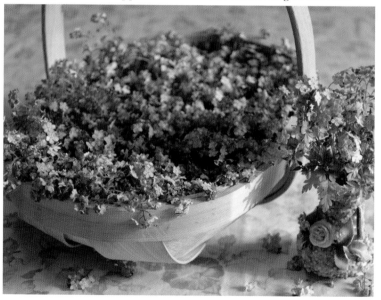

walking with his lady alongside a swollen summer river. The knight picked her a posy of forget-me-nots, but slipped and was carried away by the current. As he was drowning the knight threw the flowers to her, crying out *vergisz mein nicht*, 'forget-me-not!'

It would sound good in a German opera, but Coleridge put it in a poem, 'The Keepsake', which was published in a newspaper, and his new English name caught on (see right). We know precisely which species Coleridge was describing, because he added a footnote saying it was *M. scorpioides palustris*, water forget-me-not.

The Victorians featured forget-me-not in their language of flowers as a token of undying love.

DH Lawrence's novel *Lady Chatterley's Lover* blew such sentimentality away. The gamekeeper Mellors placed a posy of forget-me-nots on the lady's 'secret parts', as the old herbals describe them, saying *there's forget-me-nots in the right place*.

Use forget-me-not for …
Forget-me-not was known in John Parkinson's time as a source of a syrup for treating cough and 'tisicke', a consumption of the whole body as well as the lungs.

Three centuries later, Mrs Grieve (1931) confirmed the plant's affinity with the respiratory organs, notably the lower left lung.

We made a forget-me-not syrup that tasted rich, dark and densely sweet, and it did soothe the throat as it went down. Such a standard syrup was used safely for centuries to treat bronchitis, coughs, gagging and vomiting, though it is seldom used today.

Modern herbals caution that, like other members of the borage family, forget-me-not contains pyrrolizidine alkaloids, albeit in small amounts. Heat reputedly breaks them down. The flower essence is entirely safe.

Modern research
Russian clinical research (2014) has established that methyl salicylate is the principal ingredient of *M. arvensis* essential oil. This finding carries the potential for anti-inflammatory and analgesic uses of forget-me-not beyond the respiratory organs.

Clinical trials conducted on mice (2011) showed that aqueous tincture of *M. arvensis* exerts anxiolytic (anxiety-reducing) and antidepressant activity.

It was also demonstrated that essential oils of both *M. arvensis* and *M. palustris* inhibited the development of micro-organisms such as *Shigella sonnei* and *Candida albicans*. Additionally, extracts of *M. arvensis* reduced viability of *Staphylococcus aureus* and *S. faecalis*; and *M. palustris* extracts inhibited growth of *Pseudomonas aeruginosa* (2008).

Nor can I find, amid my lonely walk
By rivulet, or spring, or wet roadside
That blue and bright-eyed flowerlet of the brook,
Hope's gentle gem, the sweet Forget-me-not!
– Coleridge (1802)

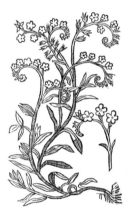

8. *Myosotis Scorpioides revens.*
Small creeping blew Mousease.

There is a Syrupe made of the juice and Sugar, by the Apothecaries of Italy and other places, which is of much account with them, to be given to those that are troubled with the cough or tisicke, which is a consumption of the whole body, as well as of the lungs.
– Parkinson (1640), with his woodcut above

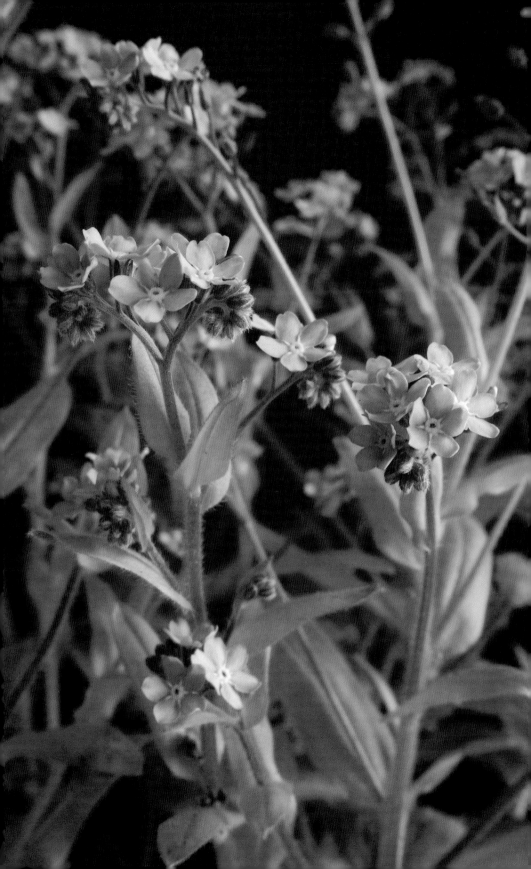

Forget-me-not flower essence
Choose a time when the flowers are at their most vibrant. Find a patch of forget-me-not growing in a peaceful sunny spot. Just sit near the plants for a while until you feel relaxed and at peace with the plants and the place. Because flower essences are based on the vibrational energy of a plant rather than its chemistry, your intention is important.

When you are ready, place a small, clear glass bowl on the ground near the plants. Fill it with about a cupful of **rain water or spring water**, then use scissors to snip off enough **flowers** to cover the surface of the water.

Leave them there for an hour or two – you can meditate on the flowers during this time, or if you prefer you can relax nearby or go for a walk while they infuse. The water will still look clear. Use a twig to lift the flowers carefully out of the water, and then use a funnel to pour the water into a bottle that is half full of **brandy.**

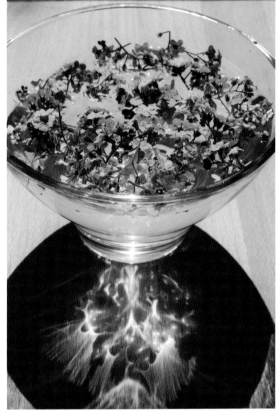

This is called your <u>mother essence</u>. Use any size of bottle you like, but a 200ml blue glass bottle works well. If any water is left over, you can drink it or water the forget-me-nots with it.

To use your mother essence, put three drops of mother essence in a 30ml dropper bottle filled with brandy. This is your <u>stock bottle</u>. With it, you can:

• put 20 drops in the bath, then soak for at least twenty minutes.
• rub directly on the skin, or mix into creams.
• put a few drops in a glass or bottle of water and sip during the day.
• make a <u>dosage bottle</u> to carry around with you, by putting three drops of stock essence into a dropper bottle containing a 50/50 brandy and water mix or pure distilled rosewater. Use several drops directly under the tongue as often as you feel you need it, or at least twice daily.

Cautions
The flower essence is completely safe, but forget-me-not contains low levels of pyrrolizidine alkaloids. Some members of this group of chemicals have caused liver damage, so the herb itself should be used with caution until more is known.

Forget-me-not essence
• grief
• clarifying
• relationships

Fumitory *Fumaria officinalis*

Papaveraceae
Poppy family

Description: Annuals, to 1m (3ft) tall, but usually shorter; many-branched stems, leaves cut fine, grey, 'smoky' from a distance; clusters of white or pink flowers with dark tips.

Habitat: Disturbed ground, fields, waysides, gardens; can grow on chalk.

Distribution: *F. officinalis* is also called common fumitory, and is widespread in the east and central British Isles, occasionally to the west; other species familiar in Europe, western Asia, widely naturalised in North America.

Related species: Three other rarer fumitories, plus six types of ramping fumitories are recorded in Britain, with much hybridisation; all share similar medicinal properties. *Dicentra formosa* (bleeding heart) and several corydalis species are also wild-growing British Fumariaceae.

Parts used: Above-ground, foliage and flowers, gathered in summer.

Common fumitory is a perky, pretty weed of field and wayside whose old name reflects its appearance as 'smoke of the earth' or *fumus terrae*. Its ancient healing reputation, especially for the liver, stomach, skin and eyes, also largely remains intact today. One modern herbalist calls it a unique gallbladder herb.

Fumitory is an important medicinal herb in both Western and Eastern traditions, and has been so since classical times. It is unusual in the sense that its principal uses – as choleretic (bile-stimulating), a tonic, a diuretic and valuable for liver, skin and eye health – have remained prominent from ancient times to today.

It was 'official', which means it was on the approved list of herbs for use by British apothecaries and doctors, in the first such list, in

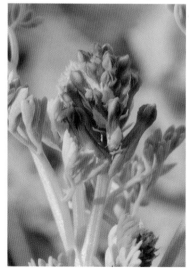

1618; and it is 'official' in the latest British list (as a choleretic) of 1996.

In 1653, the freethinking herbalist Nicholas Culpeper translated the Latin, and hence secretive, *Pharmacopoeia Londinensis* of 1618 into his own forceful English. He wrote that *Fumaria* was *cold and dry, openeth and closeth by Urine, clears the skin, opens stoppings of the Liver and Spleen, helps Rickets, Hypochondriack Melancholy, madness, frenzies, Quartan* [four-day] *Agues, loosneth the Belly*.

But what of fumitory's unusual name? Dioscorides and Pliny, some two thousand years ago, called it *kapnos*, the Greek word for smoke, because the juice of the plant made the eyes weep, as smoke does. The interesting implicit thing here is that fumitory was already in use for eye health by the Romans.

The Middle Ages had a somewhat different take. *Fumus terrae* was 'smoke of the earth', and variously meant a spontaneous growth of the plant from the ground or the 'smoky' appearance of the silvery-grey leaves from a distance. In

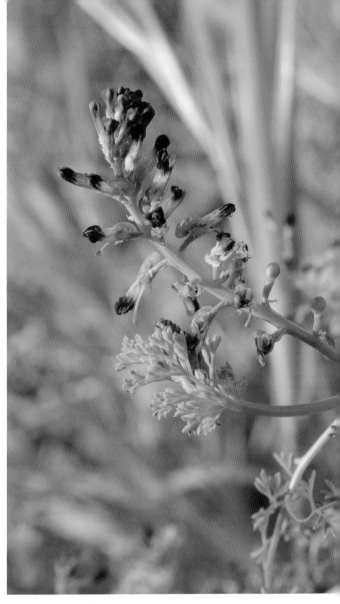

modern terms, it is possible that its sudden appearance on wayside ground or in fields is from fumitory's ability to self-fertilise.

Fumitory smoke, 'vapours of the earth', was said to drive off evil spirits, a protection against the dark side. Shakespeare had 'rank fumiter' in Lear's 'crown': *Crowned with rank fumiter and furrow-weeds/ ... and all the idle weeds that grow/ In our sustaining corn.*

'Rank' is less a comment on the plant's scent – it's not particularly bad-smelling – than the status of fumitory, and its cousins the ramping fumitories, as a weed. Its characteristic mass of finely divided leaves in older times made manual harvesting much more onerous. Anne Pratt in 1866 thought it *among the most troublesome of weeds.*

Given the long use of 'fumitory', referencing 'smoke of the earth' both in Latin and English, it's odd that English vernacular names, as collected by Grigson (1958), have no allusions to smoke. He recorded such terms as babes in the cradle, birds on the bush, God's fingers and thumbs, jam tarts, lady's lockets and wax dolls.

We offer a new name, following up on an idea from the herb writer Gabrielle Hatfield (2007): how about 'matchsticks', for the red tip on a pinky stalk, and for referencing the old allusions to smoke?

Use fumitory for ...

An important starting point is that fumitory has a reputation for safety. The European Medicines Agency monograph on fumitory (2011) collated numerous scientific studies, finding that of 710 patients tested over many years only two had experienced side effects from using the plant.

I cured a man with shocking herpes in a month with the juice and infusions of fumitory.
– Mességué (1979)

One person had suffered raised intraocular pressure and oedema, and the other a possible link to hepatitis, from using fumitory in parallel with grapevine.

The principal action of fumitory is in regulating bile flow, reducing liver stagnation and clearing liver obstructions. In particular, as Christophe Barnard points out, it keeps the sphincter of Oddi open; this muscle area affects the flow of pancreatic juices and bile into the duodenum.

Culpeper recommended boiling fumitory foliage in white wine for this 'opening' function (see quote).

The contemporary American herbalist Peter Holmes maintains that fumitory is unique among the gallbladder herbs in regulating both excess and deficiency biliary conditions (ie it is amphoteric). In the Chinese terminology Holmes uses, fumitory reduces liver qi stagnation, and as a cooling herb it modifies gallbladder damp heat.

But he adds a proviso. The array of alkaloids in fumitory has a combined dual effect, in being tonic for 8 to 10 days and then more sedative for the next 10 days.

So a patient using fumitory tea, say, for stimulating the digestion or improving bile flow would be advised to stop the treatment after 8–10 days and resume after 10 more days. Alternatively, if the more sedative, cooling range of

actions is required, a three-week treatment course of fumitory can continue uninterrupted.

Fumitory is classed in the poppy family (Papaveraceae) but is not as sedative or analgesic. Nonetheless it will effectively calm the stomach as an antispasmodic, by relaxing smooth muscle and relieving constipation; it can treat migraines linked to the stomach or liver.

It is known too as a diuretic, which stimulates urinary function and can relieve gallstones and blockages in the kidney area. It is also used in weight-loss formulas in France, but these really only cause temporary moisture loss. Also in France, fumitory maintains its older reputation as a spring tonic or 'blood cleansing' herb, flowering early and reliably for mothers to force down reluctant children as a bitterish tea.

Allied with liver function and as an aspect of excretion is the role of fumitory as a skin detoxifier. The foliage of fumitory used to be gathered, put fresh into milk and boiled for use as a lotion to lighten freckles and sunburn – as one verse put it, to 'scare the tan from Summer's cheek' (see left).

Indian fumitory (*Fumaria indica*) is known as *pitpatra*, and is a plant medicine sold in bazaars for treating skin diseases like eczema and for easing swollen joints. *Pitpatra* combined with pepper is a home treatment for ague.

Modern research

In India, Gupta et al (2012), using *F. indica* in animal studies, note anti-inflammatory actions, but not antidepressant activity; these authors also add antibacterial capacity (for *Klebsiella pneumoniae*, but not for *E. coli* or salmonella), and antifungal and antioxidant properties to the fumitory register.

A more recent Indian study (2014) on the same plant suggests a use in treating fibromyalgia.

In Iran meanwhile, a study on *F. parviflora* (2011), using the full protocol of double-blind placebo controls on 44 human patients, produced conclusive evidence of the species' effectiveness in treating hand eczema.

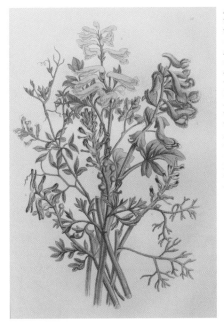

A bouquet of fumitories: common fumitory (centre) *with clockwise from lower left*: ramping fumitory, climbing corydalis, yellow fumitory, bulbous fumitory and small-flowered fumitory. Illustration from Anne Pratt, *Flowering Plants of Great Britain* Vol I (1873) pl 14, John Innes Historical Collections, courtesy of the John Innes Foundation

---

Fumitory skin lotion
As the verse (opposite) puts it, boil **fresh-gathered fumitory** in **water, milk** or **whey** to make your lotion. Put 2 handfuls of the plant into an enamel or stainless steel pan, add 1.5 cups of the chosen liquid, and boil. Simmer for 15 minutes, and leave for 15 minutes more to infuse as it cools. Pour into a jar, close and label. Store in the fridge and use freely within a week, applying morning and evening on problem skin.

Fumitory vinegar
Vinegar is a good solvent for an alkaloid-rich plant like fumitory. Choose a clean glass bottle of the appropriate size for your needs. Stuff with **dried fumitory** and fill the bottle with **white wine or apple cider vinegar**. Leave in a sunny place to macerate for a week, then strain off into another bottle. This vinegar will keep its potency for at least a year.

Dosage: 1 tablespoonful in the morning for any liver problem.

Fumitory tea
Dried fumitory is preferable for a bitter infusion: steep a heaped teaspoonful **fumitory** in **boiling water** for 5 minutes, then strain.

Fumitory skin lotion
- problem skin
- freckles
- sunburn

Fumitory vinegar
- liver stagnation
- gallbladder problems
- sphincter of Oddi dysfunction

Fumitory tea
- sluggish digestion
- lack of appetite
- spring cleanse
- liver stagnation
- gallbladder problems

Goldenrod *Solidago virgaurea*

Goldenrod is best known as a garden flower but it has a long traditional medicinal history too, among Native Americans and Elizabethan Londoners alike. It was familiar in European medicine as a wound herb and for treating kidney stones, but now offers varied and tantalising treatment possibilities.

**Asteraceae
Daisy family**

Description: Upright, untidy, with yellowish-green clusters of star-shaped, open flowers, each a small daisy; large dark green basal leaves and narrow stem leaves, variably hairy; brown seedheads.

Habitat: Invasive in wasteland and dry grassland, often on acid soils; in woodland, heathland, hedgerows and on cliffsides.

Distribution: Locally common in northern, western and southern parts of Britain and Ireland. North America. Native in Middle East.

Related species: Owing to hybridisation, the number of species is uncertain – possibly well over a hundred, most in North America. Canadian goldenrod (*Solidago canadensis*) is a common wildflower there, introduced to British Isles and an occasional alien escape.

Parts used: Flowering tops and leaves.

Goldenrod species are a familiar structural yellow presence in the wild garden, but the European goldenrod is less well known today as a powerful medicinal herb. Its genus name *Solidago* means 'to make whole or sound', a strong indication of a healing reputation; *virgaurea* is, literally, from the appearance, 'golden rod'.

The plant is also called Aaron's rod, a biblical reference to Aaron's miraculously blossoming staff, as are several other tall, wild healing perennials with spiky yellow flowers (eg agrimony and mullein).

One point of goldenrod's origin is in the Middle East, with the main European species, *S. virgaurea*, growing to 2–3 feet (0.75–1m); there are many taller native species in North America. Most abundant is Canadian goldenrod (*S. canadensis*), with feathery flower plumes up to 6 feet (2m), and a long history of Native American healing use.

Best loved of the North American varieties is sweet goldenrod (*S.*

odora) whose aniseedy aroma lends it favour as a tea herb, including in Blue Mountain Tea and formerly Liberty Tea (an ingredient of a substitute tea devised after the Boston Tea Party in 1773).

S. virgaurea had a medieval reputation as a 'woundwort' or 'Saracen's consound'. John Parkinson (1640) mentions the Arab medicine link in citing Catalan physician Arnaldus de Villanova (1235–1311), who commended its use for kidney stone and to provoke urine, as well as a sovereign wound herb to treat bruising and bleeding. Parkinson himself called it 'the best of all woundherbs'.

There was a brisk trade in imported goldenrod for such purposes in Elizabeth I's time. John Gerard (1597) notes that it once commanded a pricey half a crown an ounce in Bucklersbury, London, but after being discovered growing wild locally in Hampstead's woods its value dropped to half a crown a hundredweight.

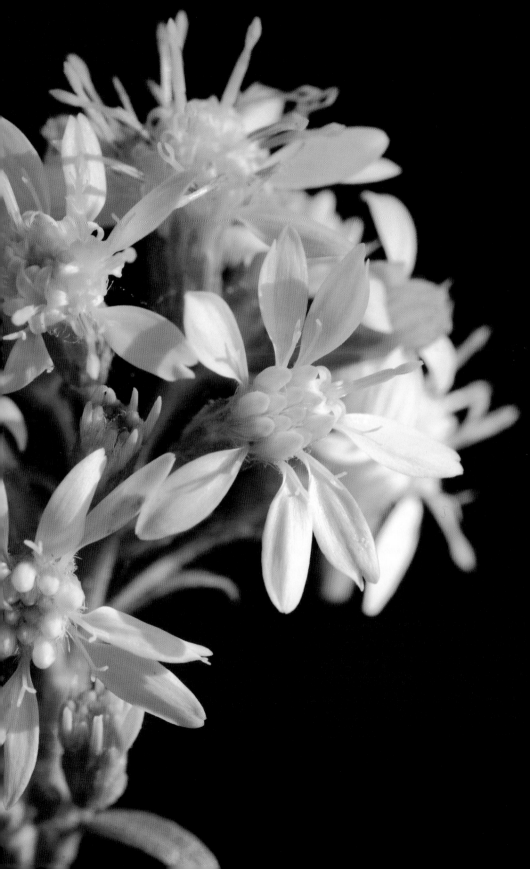

Gerard pointedly comments that this *plainly setteth foorth our inconstancie and sudden mutabilitie, esteeming no longer of any thing (how pretious soever it be) than whilest it is strange and rare*. Human psychology seems not to change much.

Use goldenrod for ...

Nicholas Culpeper's English 1653 translation of the Latin *London Dispensatory* for physicians and apothecaries captures the conventional herbal wisdom of his day for goldenrod: *hot and dry in the second degree; clenseth the Reins* [kidneys], *provokes Urin, brings away the Gravel* [calcareous deposits]; *an admirable herb for wounded people to take inwardly, stops blood &c.*

Goldenrod today is recognised among other things for its strong diuretic qualities, flushing out the system without causing loss of sodium or potassium. In Germany it is a standard kidney treatment, often preferred to pharmaceutical drugs for inflammatory diseases of the lower urinary tract. It is also used in modern irrigation therapy to prevent and break down renal and kidney calculi and gravel.

Austrian naturopath Maria Treben (1982) recommends a kidney tea made from the flowers of goldenrod mixed with species of bedstraw and deadnettle, and recounts several successful cures of otherwise intractable kidney problems. She also suggests

goldenrod as an antidepressant; the naturalist John Muir evidently agreed (see quotation).

It is regarded as a safe treatment protocol for cystitis and urethritis. It is also used as a gargle for relieving laryngitis and pharyngitis, and has been recommended as a carminative (settling the digestion).

Goldenrod has high antioxidant values – one estimate suggests seven times more than green tea. It is also antifungal, with a specific role in countering infections from *Candida albicans*, a cause of thrush of the throat or vulva.

Externally, a goldenrod ointment treated eczema, sores, ulcers and bruising; a compress made of the tea relieved muscle aches; mixed in a poultice with plantain and yarrow, it was used for burns and small wounds.

An area not highlighted in older accounts is goldenrod's value in treating upper respiratory tract disorders. This includes influenza, chronic and acute catarrh; it is 'official' for catarrh in the *British Herbal Pharmacopoeia* (1996).

The treatment would generally be a tea of the dried or fresh flowering tops and leaves. Native Americans chewed goldenrod flowers for sore throats, and also made a tea for reducing fevers. Interestingly, asthma is a condition efficiently treated by goldenrod flowers. This is despite an undeserved but persistent reputation for causing summer allergies. In North America the blame for these has been reallocated to ragweed (*Ambrosia* spp.) whose flowering season overlaps with that of goldenrod. Ragweed pollen is thought to cause over 90% of allergies in the US summer months.

Modern research
Goldenrod contains plentiful tannins, and is now recognised as an anti-inflammatory. It has been compared to diclofenac, a proprietary NSAID used for treating rheumatoid arthritis.

What is increasingly recognised (eg 2004 research) is the 'rather complex' spectrum of goldenrod's phytotherapeutic actions. It is known to be anti-inflammatory, antimicrobial, diuretic, antispasmodic and analgesic, an unusual combination of 'virtues' that offers tantalising research directions.

For example, it has been shown to be cardioprotective in rats (2014) and to treat prostatic cancer in mice (2002). Human trials are awaited.

The rhizome of a Chilean goldenrod (*S. chilensis*), sometimes called Brazilian arnica, produced (2008) a marked anti-inflammatory response in mice, by inhibiting both proinflammatory mediators and leucocyte infiltration. The same plant relieved symptoms and pain of human lumbago (2009).

Research also confirms goldenrod's anti-*Candida* credentials: a 2012 study using *S. virgaurea* showed effectiveness against two key virulence factors of *C. albicans*: the yeast-hyphal transition phase and biofilm formation.

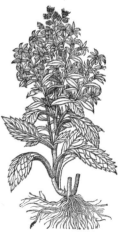

2 Virga aurea serratis foliis.
Golden Rod with densed leaves.

Goldenrod, woodcut, Parkinson, *Theatrum Botanicum* (1640)

Caution
Goldenrod species freely hybridise, which may lead to variations in wild-gathered species' phytochemical actions. Previous herbal interpretations of goldenrod as variously 'warming' or 'cooling' may be an instance of such species variation. The general actions of goldenrod species are similar and interchangeable, but herbal users should be aware of potential variation.

Goldenrod syrup
• sore throats
• coughs
• urinary tract inflammation
• cystitis
• urethritis
• irritable bowel

Goldenrod syrup
Harvest **goldenrod** while it is in flower in the summer. Place in a pan and cover with **water**, bringing slowly to the boil. Simmer gently for a few minutes, then remove from heat. Cover the saucepan with a lid and leave overnight to infuse.

Strain off the liquid and return to a clean pan. Add 200g **sugar** to every 250ml of liquid, and bring to the boil. Stir until all the sugar has dissolved. Warm your bottles, then pour the syrup in, cap and label.

Dosage: 1 teaspoonful 3 or 4 times a day, especially for children.

If you like your syrups less sweet, try adding **fresh lemon juice** when you add the sugar. Use the juice of 1 lemon per 500 ml of liquid.

Greater celandine *Chelidonium majus*

Papaveraceae
Poppy family

Description: Common perennial, 1m (3ft) tall, with relatively small lemon yellow flowers, each of four petals, on top of profuse, branched lime-green foliage, with rounded leaves; distinctive orange sap and long thin seed capsules.

Habitat: Disturbed waste land, banks, hedgerows, walls near human habitation; may often be escapes from old physic gardens.

Distribution: Native to temperate Europe, Eurasia, introduced to eastern and western North America.

Related species: No direct relative, and certainly not Lesser celandine (a buttercup). Is in a genus with but one species. Welsh poppy (*Meconopsis cambrica*) is another British yellow-flowered poppy with four petals.

Parts used: Whole plant, including orange sap (which stains but is washable) and roots.

Greater celandine might be taken for a large, leafy mustard topped by small yellow flowers, but it is in fact a poppy. Like its *Papaver* cousins, it has a stem latex and a complex array of alkaloids/enzymes, which underlie both its long-known herbal virtues and regulatory concern about its potential toxicity.

Greater celandine has a long tradition of use in European and Chinese folk medicine (as *Bai qu cai*) as a liver and bile herb, with external applications in eye and skin health. In energetic terms, notes American herbalist Peter Holmes, its leafy green appearance with yellow flowers suggests a liver remedy, but he suggests it is better understood as *a warming cardiovascular stimulant as much as a hepatic stimulant*.

Thus, it acts to restore coronary circulation and relieve sharp chest pains (angina) brought on by over-exertion when there is inadequate blood supply to the heart. It also has an antispasmodic action, which works to relieve colic in the intestines, wheezing and coughing in the lungs, and asthma.

Greater celandine's ability to soothe bronchial spasms led to its use in treating whooping

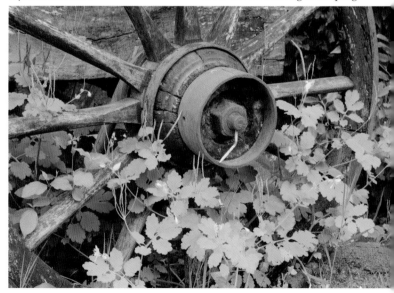

cough and bronchitis, especially in China. Holmes notes there was no equal to it in the Chinese pharmacopoeia, and it was long used in Chinese hospitals.

Use greater celandine for …
Greater celandine's stimulant effect extends to use as a bitter tea or tincture to promote sweating (as a diaphoretic), urination (as a diuretic) and irregular menstruation (as an emmenagogue). Being a uterine stimulant means it should not be taken during pregnancy.

Arising from these properties greater celandine is useful to help the body sweat out colds, flu and fatigue; relieve limb and ankle swelling (oedema or dropsy); and as a useful ingredient in gout or arthritis treatments.

Better known is the way the plant promotes bile flow (as a chloretic), alleviates the pain of gallstones, and reduces liver congestion and any related migraine headaches (as an analgesic). It has been regarded as a jaundice (hepatitis) herb, but in excess can be damaging to the liver.

British herbalist Julian Barker makes the important point that the active alkaloid and other constituents of greater celandine and their interactions vary greatly; the plant product, fresh or dried, and however extracted, is not stable, with a short shelf life; and although safe within therapeutic

limits it is potentially toxic. Dosage is key here, and any internal use of this plant should be within limits recommended by a practitioner.

It is good practice to take a break of several days in treatment after two weeks. Homeopathic use is an alternative. French herbalist Maurice Mességué recommended footbaths using greater celandine.

A still-popular use of the plant's orange sap or caustic juice is to treat corns, warts, veruccas, herpes and other skin eruptions. Old names for greater celandine, such as tetterwort (tetters are variously ringworm, herpes and eczema) and felonwort (a felon is a whitlow, an abscess of the nail), testify to folkloric usage.

We now know the sap contains protein-dissolving enzymes that destroy malignant viruses on the skin. This suggests the strength of the sap and any washes derived from it, and underlines why application should be restricted to the infected / inflamed area and not broken skin or open wounds.

One French herbalist calls external use of the plant 'irreplaceable', and claims *it will generally cause ugly cutaneous excrescences to vanish within eight days*.

A recent proponent of the use of the orange sap of greater celandine for the eyes is the Austrian herbalist Maria Treben. Her 1982 book

It wipes out herpes, deals with ringworm, literally melts away warts and corns and speeds up the healing of ulcers. … As a foot-bath, it regularizes women's periods, and brings them on after an abnormal stoppage.
– Mességué (1979)

… clearly, much of the story of this plant remains to be told.
– Hatfield (2007)

Caution
Greater celandine should not be taken internally during pregnancy. Its internal use is restricted in some countries.

records she applied it in drop doses on patients with cataracts, but also for her own healthy but tired eyes. At the end of a long day, when writing letters, she would wet a leaf, squeeze it, then apply the juice – *It is as if a mist is lifted from my eyes,* she wrote.

Our own view is that given the caustic strength of the raw sap it ought to be diluted if used, and under advice from your herbalist.

Modern research
Greater celandine has a mixed reputation in cancer treatment, specifically for skin and stomach cancer. This is not new: William Langham, in 1578, proposed it in an external skin cancer treatment: [For] *Kanker, wash it well with wine or vineger, and then apply the iuice of the hearbe and roots thereof.*

The European Medicines Agency has a 40-page assessment (2009) of greater celandine, and confirms its anti-tumour effects *in vitro* (on rats and mice) as 'very promising' but *in vivo* studies on mice are at an early stage. More human research, inevitably, is called for.

The same EMA report also notes a variety of dose-dependent antiviral, antioxidant, antimicrobial and anti-inflammatory effects of the plant reported in ongoing research (eg candida, herpes, RNA polio virus and *E. coli*).

This 'official' evidence is positive for such wider uses of greater celandine, a fact that should not be overlooked when considering the downside – that in some people liver toxicity results from taking it in treatments, with symptoms of fullness, gastro-enteritis, diarrhoea and other disturbances.

Because internal use of greater celandine is restricted to practitioners, we are only recommending it for external use.

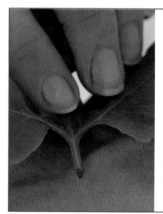

Greater celandine sap
The sap can be used any time there are green leaves of lesser celandine available, but there is generally more sap produced in warmer weather.

Break off a leaf and allow the yellowy-orange sap to emerge from the stem. Carefully apply the sap to warts or other unbroken skin blemishes. Repeat frequently, and you should see results within days.

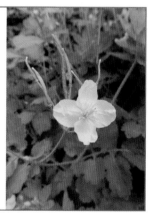

Ground elder *Aegopodium podagraria*

'Love your weeds' is an invocation that might stretch patience and credulity in the case of ground elder. Yet a positive case can be made for this garden pestilence as a traditional gout and anti-inflammatory treatment, a forage food, and most intriguingly as a potential player in the struggle against kidney and liver disease and metabolic syndrome.

**Apiaceae
Carrot family**

Description: Perennial, with hairless, hollow stems, rhizomes and white stolons; pinnate leaves, resembling but unrelated to elder; attractive umbels of white flowers, to 1m (3ft).

Habitat: Gardens predominantly, also waysides, disturbed ground, woodland margins.

Distribution: Native to Central Europe, Eurasia; introduced to Britain, Western Europe, North America and other temperate regions.

Related species: There are up to eight Aegopodiums worldwide but this is the common Eurasian species.

Parts used: Leaves, roots.

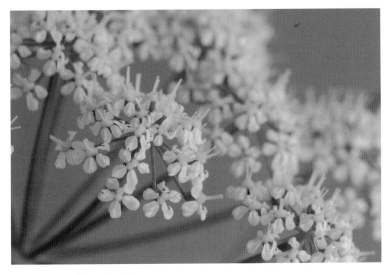

Extreme gardener Stephen Barstow describes ground elder as 'perhaps the most invasive widespread introduced plant in gardens in Europe'. So why include a terrorist of the borders in a book about wayside plants?

We had not often seen ground elder outside a garden context until summer 2015, when we visited Loughcrew, in Westmeath, Ireland. There, along a quiet road, a few hundred yards from the nearest house, was a mass of

flowering ground elder. It was not just the dominant Apiaceae but the dominant plant, outmuscling nettles, herb robert, cleavers and other vigorous settlers.

So, yes, ground elder is largely a plant of gardens, but also waysides, churchyards and other disturbed habitats, sometimes as a garden discard. Its roots are said to grow up to a metre a year, and it needs only a few millimetres of root to clone itself, just as woodbine and couch grass

I have known a quantity of the roots and leaves boiled soft together, and applied to the hip in sciatica, keeping a fresh quantity hot to renew the other, as it grew cold, and I have seen great good effect from it.
– Hill (1812)

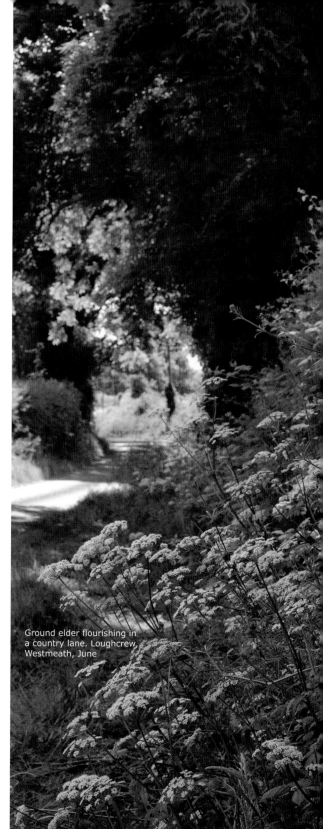

do. Incidentally, these other two invasives also have long-standing herbal uses, and we argue for ground elder in this respect. One English sufferer calls it Grelda, a 'seemingly immortal witch-weed', and Matthew's mother refused to take any rooted plants from our garden because we have ground elder. It is banned, declared toxic, in many states in the US and elsewhere.

The problem, unfortunately, is not new. In his lifetime John Gerard was as well known for his Holborn flower garden as for his *Herball* (1597). He writes with resignation: *Herbe Gerard groweth of itself in gardens without setting or sowing and is so fruitful in its increase that when it hath once taken roote, it will hardly be gotten out againe, spoiling and getting every yeare more ground, to the annoying of better herbe.*

Full of self-belief as he was, Gerard was not naming the plant after himself. St Gerard of Toul (935–994) was the patron saint of gout sufferers, and ground elder was used, even before the saint, as a home remedy for gout.

The plant had the medieval name bishopweed, perhaps because of the link between gout and the drinking habits of the higher clergy, or because ground elder was a monastic plant – useful both in the kitchen as a spring vegetable and in the infirmary for compresses and teas to relieve gout, rheumatism and sciatica.

Ground elder flourishing in a country lane. Loughcrew, Westmeath, June

The species name *podagraria* is from *podagra*, or gout, so goutweed as a common name has a direct link to its observed use. The generic name *Aegopodium*, from words meaning foot and goat, is probably from the shape of the young leaves looking somewhat like the foot of a goat. American forager 'Wildman' Steve Brill believes goutweed has no effect on gout and that the common name is a corruption of the older goatweed. Few seem to agree.

The plant is thought to have had its origin in the Caucasus, Ukraine and Central Asia, spreading westwards by planting (yes, some people do this), clonal reproduction and seed dispersal (an old name is jack-jump-about).

When it arrived in Britain is moot. Some argue for a Roman introduction, others for the monastic period. Archaeological evidence from Denmark shows it was there in Iron Age times, but no similar pre-Roman discoveries have been made in Britain. Perhaps several reintroductions?

Coming up to date, Stephen Barstow is a pioneer collector and grower of unusual edible plants. What is remarkable is that he gardens near Trondheim, Norway, that is, north of the Arctic Circle. The Gulf Stream warms this area but the growing season is still very short. One of the plants he champions is ground elder, and he wants to stop its 'persecution'.

So Stephen has formed the Friends of Ground Elder as a Facebook group, with the goal of ending the chemical warfare on the plant and putting a long-overdue positive case for its use. It may be an uphill battle, but we're backing him.

Use ground elder for …
So is goutweed good for gout? To Parkinson 'goutewort', is not named 'at randome', but *upon good experience to helpe the cold Goute and Sciatica and other cold griefs.*

This finding is widely replicated, with ground elder tea made from the leaves drunk or used externally to soak a poultice or fomentation for treating gout, sciatica, piles and diarrhoea. Julie found drinking the tea beneficial for her own sciatica one year.

The same remedy is a traditional wound herb, used for soothing burns, stings, bites and wounds externally. Tinctures are less used traditionally, though the German herbalist Tabernaemontanus (1520–90) liked to cook the plant in wine for similar purposes.

Such older medicinal uses remain available. What of cooking ground elder, as a spring green or eating raw? One forager's soup and quiche are *all the tastier from being made from the bodies of an enemy.*

We rather like its raw, anise-like taste and texture when fresh, but a little goes a long way, especially in a salad. We disguised the effect

They [ground elder patches] don't just occupy the places between the cultivated flowers. They subvert them, insinuating their white subterranean tendrils, as supple as earthworms, around and through any root system in their way.
– Mabey (2010)

I wouldn't do without it as a vegetable and I use it frequently in spring over a 6–8 week period when the fresh young growth is available. I also use it later in the summer where it regenerates after I scythe the areas where it still grows in my forest garden.
– Barstow (2014)

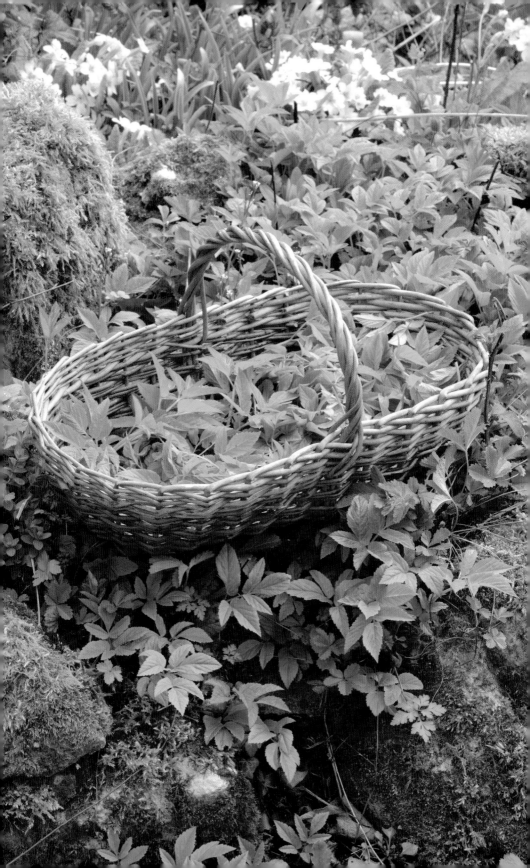

in a pleasant-tasting frittata and a sag paneer, and other cooks have used the leaves in pizza, curry and borscht. Another possibility is drying the leaves to a powder for a green smoothie, or trying the white stolons in a cooked form.

Modern research

Tovchiga et al in Ukraine trialled ground elder tincture in rat uric acid metabolism and suppression of inflammation (2014). The tincture showed protective action in kidney function, such as reducing proteinuria and hyperazotemia, and protecting the liver from carbon tetrachloride-induced hepatitis. Further, the tincture's hypoglycaemic property was found to be beneficial in metabolic syndrome treatment.

These are potentially key discoveries for application of new pharmaceuticals but also for herbal use of ground elder in these problematic areas. The next stage will be human trials.

Other research has shown that ground elder root has a type of supra-molecular protein, a lectin (1987); and that mature flowers contain falcarindiol, with proven COX-1 activity (2007).

The combination of [A. podagraria's] hypoglycemic, nephroprotective, hepatoprotective, antiinflammatory properties as well as ability to normalize uric acid metabolism can be of great value in metabolic syndrome treatment.
– Tovchiga (2014)

Ground elder frittata

This is a vegan version that we often eat, made with all sorts of wild greens, but ground elder is our favourite.

Preheat oven to 175°C (350°F). Put in a blender: 1 cup **gram flour** (chick pea flour), 2 cups **water**, ½ teaspoon **salt**, 1 or 2 peeled cloves of **garlic** and 1 teaspoon **turmeric powder.** Blend until smooth, then set aside to rest while you sauté the vegetables.

Put 1 tablespoon **olive oil** in a large skillet. Add sliced **mushrooms**, chunks of **cooked potato**, and a couple of handfuls of chopped **ground elder leaves**.

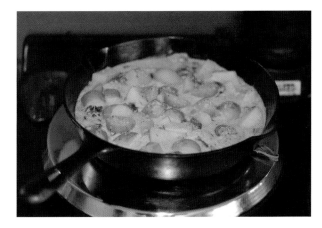

When the vegetables are cooked, pour the blended liquid over them and cook until the edges of the batter are set, then transfer into the preheated oven for 15 minutes. The frittata should be set, and gently browned on top.

Slice and serve warm.

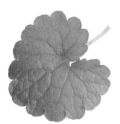

Ground ivy *Glechoma hederacea*

A common European and American perennial wildflower, ground ivy was once, and could be again, a home medicinal. It is best known as an expectorant catarrh-clearing herb and for head and kidney issues, but research is underlining its value as an anti-inflammatory, antioxidant and antibacterial.

Lamiaceae
Deadnettle family

Description: Low-growing creeping perennial, 20–30cm (8–12in) high. Crinkly, heart-shaped, opposite leaves; gently hairy square stems, each with 2–4 rich purple flowers in whorls, with 'Lamiaceae lip' and musty smell; underground stolons (creeping runners) can be a metre/yard long.

Habitat: Damp semi-shade in woods, scrub, hedgerows, grassland.

Distribution: Very common throughout British Isles, except west of Ireland and Scottish Highlands; widespread in northern and central Europe, east to Siberia and temperate Asia. Introduced by early settlers to North America, now common in most states.

Related species: Ground ivy is the only western species in the Glechoma genus; *G. longituba* is used as a medicinal in China. Unrelated to common ivy (*Hedera helix*).

Parts used: Above-ground parts.

Ground ivy, like many old country herbs, acquired a cluster of affectionate names. Some refer to its appearance, like cats foot (for the circular leaves); robin run in the hedge or creeping charlie in the US (for the spreading stolons); and blue runner (for the flowers).

Other names reflect its long period of use, from the Anglo-Saxons to the Tudors, as the main bitter herb for brewing and clarifying ale. It was alehoof ('hoof' meaning herb) or tunhoof ('tun', meaning the verb to brew or the cask itself), while from the French *guiller* (to brew) it became gill.

Gill was also a measure of liquid, still taught in primary school in Matthew's time – four gills make one (British) pint. The word, as Mrs Grieve mentions, also meant 'girl', so ground ivy sometimes was hedgemaid or hay maiden.

Interestingly, for a plant that was also a popular medicinal, it attracted few overtly healing names, field balm being one. And, as Geoffrey Grigson pointed out in 1958, the English 'ground

ivy' itself was a 'poor name'. A version of *Hedera terrestris*, or Old English 'eorthifig', ground ivy has no relationship with ivy other than being a vine.

Use ground ivy for…
Thomas Bartram's well-regarded herbal reference book gives 'catarrh' as a keynote descriptor for ground ivy; we prefer 'clarity'. Combining the two ideas, wherever there is congestion trust ground ivy to clear it!

Ground ivy is expectorant – indeed, this is the sole function attributed to it in the latest *British Herbal Pharmacopoeia* (1996) – hence anti-catarrhal, or phlegm-clarifying, if you prefer. Bartram notes that the catarrh can be bronchial or nasal.

Ground ivy was widely used in tea form for 'inveterate coughs' and consumption (pulmonary tuberculosis), and remains highly effective in lung conditions.

Hildegard von Bingen (1098–1179) believed that ground ivy removed bad humours from the head. We

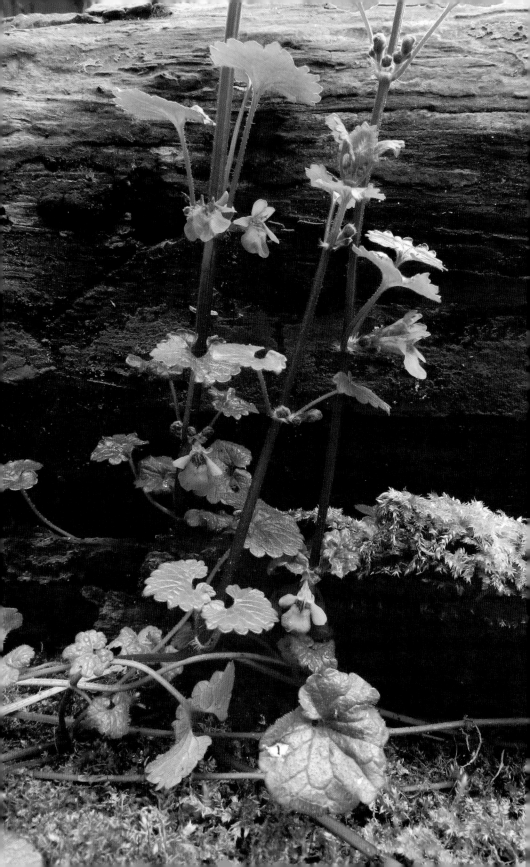

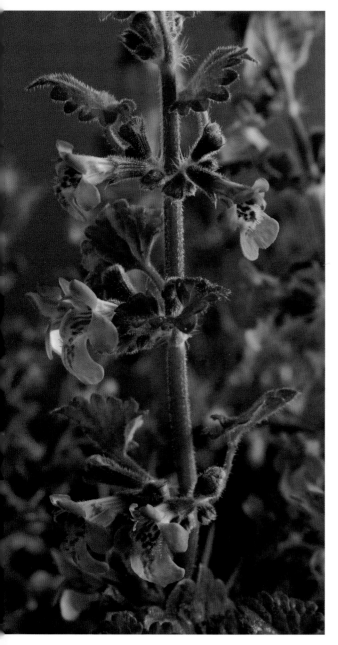

agree, and view ground ivy as the equal of rosemary as a 'head herb'.

Ground ivy is an ancient, safe herbal treatment for tinnitus, sinusitis and 'glue ear'. It makes a soothing wash for the eyes, or can be powdered and snuffed to clear the nose. As a compress it can be applied to the forehead for migraines or on 'black eyes'.

It has been useful for pain relief in toothache: William Langham in 1577 suggested: *Boile it with ginger in wine and hold thereof in thy mouth.*

It is also an 'important astringent', says Bartram, for the stomach, intestines and colon. It has a special affinity for the kidneys and bladder, as befits a diuretic herb. Poor kidney function can lead to chest congestion and breathing issues, areas ground ivy supports.

Bringing the astringent and anti-inflammatory qualities together, a recent survey recommends ground ivy for dyspepsia, gastritis, diarrhoea, irritable bowel syndrome, piles, cystitis and abdominal colic.

Another former use was as a tea to counteract 'painter's colic' or the lead poisoning from paint.

Modern research
The antimicrobial power of ground ivy was shown in 2011, when it tested as the most toxic to bacteria of the Lamiaceae species in bactericidal studies.

It was shown (2006) to inhibit nitrous oxide in conditions of macrophage-mediated inflammation, suggesting use in metabolic disease.

A traditional Japanese tea, *kakidoushi-cha*, made from *Glechoma hederacea* var. *grandis*, was found (2013) to inhibit the enzyme xanthine oxidase, making the tea protective in liver and gout issues.

Korean research (2014), testing *G. hederacea* for osteoclastogenesis, found potential for the plant's use in treating bone disorders such as osteoporosis and rheumatoid arthritis; turmeric (curcumin) and *Angelica sinensis* have shown similar potential.

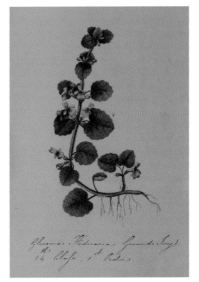

Ground ivy, from Anna Sophia Clitherow's Watercolour Sketchbooks, c.1804–1815, John Innes Historical Collections, courtesy of the John Innes Foundation

... the juice dropped into the eares doth wonderfully helpe the noyse and singing of them, and helpeth their hearing that is decayed.
– Parkinson (1640)

Meigrim [migraine], anoint the forehead and nostrels with the iuice, vinegar and oyle, or stampe [crush] the leaues with the white of an egge, & apply it.
– Langham (1577)

As a medicine useful in pulmonary complaints, where a tonic for the kidneys is required, it would appear to possess peculiar suitability, and is well adapted to all kidney complaints.
– Grieve (1931)

Harvesting ground ivy
Ground ivy is most aromatic in spring and summer (the smell varies by location), but the leaves stay green and are available most of the year.

Ground ivy clari-tea
Heat **water** (or wine or beer if you prefer) in a small saucepan, and add a few sprigs of fresh **ground ivy** for each cup of liquid when the liquid comes to the boil. Remove from heat, cover and allow to steep for 5 or 10 minutes. Strain and use the liquid.

Drink hot with honey or other sweetener, to taste. This drink once had the country name of gill tea. Most people find it has a satisfying taste and feels comforting to the throat. We mostly make ground ivy tea in the spring when it is in flower, but the leaves can be used anytime.

It can be reheated or drunk cold, as many cups a day as can be tolerated. The cold liquid can also be the basis of a compress: soak a cloth in the juice and apply to bruises, abscesses, headaches and sore eyes to take out the heat.

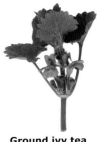

Ground ivy tea
- clears the head
- clears the mind
- congestion
- catarrh & phlegm
- stuffy nose
- tinnitus
- sinusitis

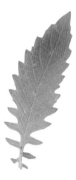

Gypsywort *Lycopus europaeus*

From an apparently disreputable past, gypsywort has now become a valued medicinal. Along with its American cousin, bugleweed, it has the specific ability to treat hyperthyroidism, or Graves' disease, safely and reduce the associated racing heartbeat and anxiety. Other benefits also repay a second look.

**Lamiaceae
Deadnettle family**

Description:
Perennial, to 1m
(3ft); erect stature,
with opposite jagged-
toothed leaves; in
summer bears tiny
white flower whorls,
with purple spots, in
the leaf axils; grows in
massed colonies.

Habitat: Wetlands,
whether ditches, pond
sides, riverbanks, damp
woodland.

Distribution: Native
to Europe and Turkey;
common in England
and Wales south of
Yorkshire, western
Scotland, and scattered
elsewhere. Introduced
in North America.

Related species:
Other Lycopus species,
native to North
America, include
Virginia bugleweed
(*L. virginicus*),
American bugleweed
(*L. americanus*) and
'Chinese' bugleweed (*L.
lucidus*).

Parts used: Leaves,
which are stronger
medicinally than the
roots, and above-
ground parts.

Gypsywort seems to have always been an outsider. In ancient times its deeply serrated leaf was likened to a wolf's foot (literally *Lycopus*) – hinting at transgressive as well as fanciful. And does the 'gypsy' in the plant's common name signify uncertain fears and prejudices about 'others'?

The first English account, in Henry Lyte's herbal (1578), describes how *the rogues and runagates, which name themselves Egyptians* [Gypsies], *do colour themselves blacke with this herbe*. The charge was elaborated in later accounts that travelling Romanies would dye their faces with the herb to look more exotic and then proceed to con the locals with magic and fortune-telling.

A more generous, but unrecorded, scenario would be that the Gypsies might have used the dye for their clothes rather than their faces, or perhaps have been the first to use and convey the health-giving properties of the plant (and hence give it 'wort' status).

English herbalist Julian Barker notes that in North America the

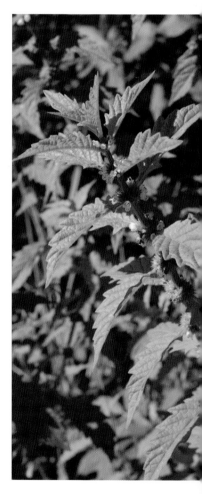

Native American peoples used their local Lycopus species as medicine and ate the roots.

Gypsywort's closest medicinal relative is the Virginia bugleweed (*Lycopus virginicus*) of the eastern US, which is thought to be slightly more bioactive, and has another common name, gypsyweed, that suggests similarity. This is the species most often used today on both sides of the Atlantic.

Two other American species are valued herbally, namely American bugleweed or water horehound (*Lycopus americanus*), and 'Chinese' bugleweed (*L. lucidus*). All the Lycopus species are perennials, need a wetland habitat and have comparable medicinal uses.

Gypsywort has little aroma and only two stamens, though it does share the square stems, opposite leaves, bunched flower whorls and running stolons of its mint cousins like lemon balm and motherwort with which it is often prescribed.

Use gypsywort for...
Bugleweed is the form of *Lycopus* most used commercially by herbalists on both sides of the Atlantic, but rather than importing it, British herbalists might well reconsider their native gypsywort.

Bugleweed itself was far from an outsider, and was mainstream medicine in 19th-century America, being included for a while in the *U.S. Pharmacopoeia.*

It was recommended at that time as nerve-calming and sedative, anti-haemorrhagic, anti-tussive (for coughs and lung problems), for urinary problems and as a mild narcotic that was safer than foxglove (digitalis). Such uses remain valid.

But what made *Lycopus* specifically valuable was the early 20th-century extension of its therapeutic range to include overactive thyroid and the associated racing heartbeat. Today bugleweed and gypsywort are the go-to herbs for treating hyperthyroidism, usually caused by Graves' (or Basedow) disease.

Graves' is an auto-immune condition that largely affects women from middle age onwards. Sufferers experience raised levels of iodine and thyroid-stimulating hormone (TSH), which the plants safely lower while also maintaining thyroid gland health.

Graves' is typified by accelerated heart rate, palpitations and related anxiety, along with goitre of the eyes, sometimes called 'wild staring'. Bugleweed and gypsywort taken as leaf tea or tincture can reduce these alarming symptoms, often given with lemon balm and motherwort to deepen the soothing and sedative effect.

Note that while small and regular doses of the plants improve the symptom picture for hyperthyroidism, its fundamental

... one of the mildest and best narcotics in existence. It acts somewhat like Digitalis, and lowers the pulse, without producing any of its bad effects nor accumulating in the system.
– Rafinesque (1828)

... one of the precious few thyroid inhibitors.
– Holmes (2006)

Traditional herbal treatment for hyperthyroidism provides us with one of the best examples of a condition for which a definite specific exists. This is Lycopus virginicus or L. europaeus, commonly known as bugleweed.
– Hoffmann (2003)

Caution: Bugleweed and gypsywort are safe to take long-term, but pregnant and lactating women are advised to suspend their use. Prolonged hormone imbalances, including TSH, should be referred to a practitioner.

Where there is pre-existing thyroid gland enlargement or weak thyroid function, *Lycopus* is contra-indicated. In one case in the literature high levels of *Lycopus* caused thyroid enlargement.

The mint-like character of gypsywort's flowering tops

causes may be much harder to treat. Some authors describe the condition as genetic and incurable. Yet the plants have much to offer Graves' sufferers in quality of life. The same could be said for other herbal virtues the plants have been shown to possess, in reducing internal bleeding, such as heavy menstruation, calming tubercular and bronchial spasms, and being excellent relievers of indigestion.

Modern research
There has been experimental confirmation on Lycopus for its thyroid effects (2006) and the reduction in TSH levels (1994). Chinese research (2013), using *L. lucidus* on rabbits, showed cardiotonic effects, confirming traditional uses. Korean research on the same plant (2008) showed its leaves suppress high glucose-induced vascular inflammation.

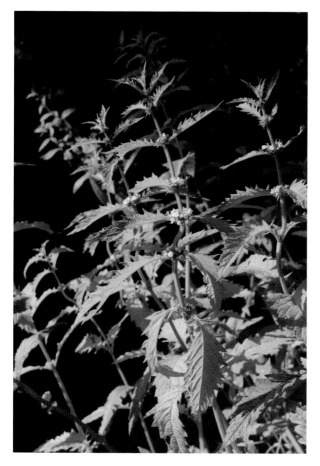

Gypsywort tincture
Pick gyspywort when it is flowering in late summer. Chop it into one inch pieces, and place in a jar. Pour in enough vodka to cover it, then put the lid on and shake to release any air bubbles, topping up if necessary.

Put the jar in a dark place for about a month, shaking every few days. When the colour has gone out of the leaves, strain off the liquid and bottle it.

Dosage: half to one teaspoonful 3 times a day. It may be necessary to take a dose more frequently initially.

If you have an overactive thyroid, it is a serious condition requiring professional help and advice from your GP and a practising herbalist.

Gypsywort is often used in combination with lemon balm (*Melissa officinalis*) and motherwort (*Leonurus cardiaca*) for palpitations and over-active thyroid.

Heather, ling *Calluna vulgaris*
Bell heather *Erica cinerea*

Heather is much more than a pretty moorland scene on a Scottish shortbread tin. Historically, the two main species were a vital part of everyday life in many acid-soil upland areas, especially Scotland, and still have a significant economic role. Never accepted as 'official' medicine, heather's popular herbal uses have largely disappeared, but research is confirming traditional knowledge and opening up intriguing possibilities.

As well as the heathers themselves, the heather family contains many useful and decorative acidic soil-loving shrubs and smaller plants, such as rhododendrons, azaleas, vacciniums (including the fruitful cranberry, bilberry, blueberry and cowberry), bearberries and one tree, the strawberry tree.

The main heather species are subdivided into one Calluna species – ling or heather (*Calluna vulgaris*) – and at least ten Ericas, or heaths, including bell heather (*Erica cinerea*) and cross-leaved heath (*E. tetralix*).

Ling and bell heather are dominant in their heathland habitats; indeed they give their name to it. There are minor botanical variations, but the difference between them is observed best when they grow together: the swathes of magenta-purple flowers are bell heather, and the delicate mauve is ling.

Herbally, they have seldom been distinguished and have overlapping medicinal uses. Bell heather, however, makes for a stronger, darker honey, while ling honey is more viscous.

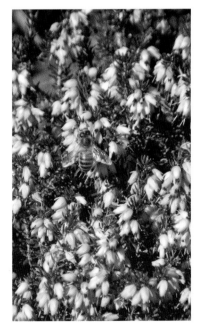

Ericaceae
Heather family

Description: Both species are evergreen shrubs growing to about 60cm tall. Heather or ling, *Calluna vulgaris*, has small purplish pink flowers appearing in late summer; bell heather or heath, *Erica cinerea*, has larger, brighter magenta pot shaped flowers over a slightly longer season, from May to October.

Habitat: Heath, moor, open woodland and bog, mainly poor acid, peaty or rocky soils.

Distribution: Widespread in the upland and moorland British Isles, especially to the north and west, and in the south. *Calluna vulgaris* is introduced in US.

Related species: Cross-leaved heath (*E. tetralix*) is the third main species, with similar distribution to bell heather but prefers wetter soils. Dorset heath (*E. ciliaris*) and Cornish heath (*E. vagans*) have restricted local habitats.

Parts used: Medicinally, the flowering tops, gathered in summer, used fresh or dried.

Heather or ling

Heather, from Anna Sophia Clitherow's Watercolour Sketchbooks, c.1804–1815, John Innes Historical Collections, courtesy of the John Innes Foundation

Scottish heather ale, after centuries of neglect, is currently back in favour, sold under the Gaelic name *fraoch*. The heather takes the hops role in brewing, mixed with malted barley and bog myrtle.

The Victorian botanist Anne Pratt noted that *those who have few resources learn to make the most of them*. This applies aptly to the way heather was an indispensable part of moorland life. It was a foundation for roads and tracks; it made walls and thatch, ropes, baskets and fish traps; it could tan leather; it was a food for domestic animals in winter; it made springy but comfortable bedding.

Calluna, interestingly, is not classical but from an 18th-century reclassification of the heathers. The name means 'brush', and may refer to bunches of ling made into besoms or informal brushes; or it might reflect medicinal use for the digestive and urinary tracts.

'Ling' is thought to derive from an Anglo-Saxon term for 'fire'. The young shoots of ling are the red grouse's favourite food. In modern economic terms, 'grouse moors' are valuable assets – ironically, just as moorland, the former symbol of a poor but self-sufficient peasantry, is being lost to various forms of 'development'.

The traditional communal reliance on heather may reflect a bygone age, but can be adapted by today's camping buff. Heather bunches make a good base for a sleeping bag; dead stems can fuel a campfire and young plant tips flavour tea – sweetened with heather honey. After your meal, clean your enamel plates with strands of heather. If it's raining, sit dry in your tent making a heather basket for ripe bilberries!

One final tip for wet walks is to follow the magenta clumps of bell heather as a marker of dry ground, which it prefers, amid more boggy areas preferred by cross-leaved heath (also known as bog heath).

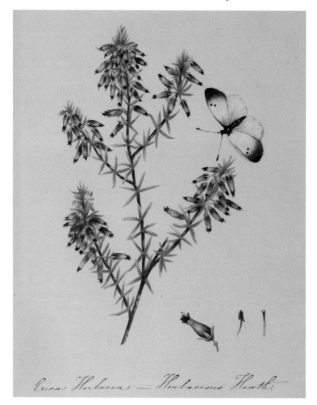

Erica Herbacea — Herbaceous Heath

Bell heather and gorse,
Dartmoor, August

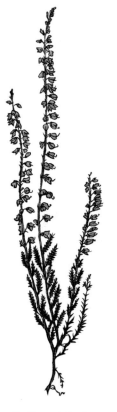

Heather, painting by
Rudolf Koch and Fritz
Kredel (1929), John
Innes Historical Collec-
tions, courtesy of the
John Innes Foundation

Use heather for …

As a medicinal, heather has classical origins in the 1st- and 2nd-century AD writings of Dioscorides and Galen, and the Erica family has been long known for its effectiveness in treating conditions of the urinary tract.

Bearberry, *Uva ursi*, is a close relative, found in Scotland, and is currently prescribed by herbalists for cystitis, prostate issues, inflammatory bladder and urinary stone or gravel. Heather could be a local, plentiful alternative.

Heather is antiseptic and diuretic for the digestive and urinary tracts, and takes these actions into easing the pain of nephritis, gout, arthritis and rheumatism.

Heather tea can be made from dried or fresh plants. Robert Burns called it 'moorland tea'. Heather tincture and distilled water are equally effective medicinally, and any of these forms can be applied in heather poultices or liniments. A heather bath can ease chilblains.

The original name *Erica* was linked in classical writings to 'breaking' in the sense of an internal stone. Parkinson reported the Italian botanist Matthiolus (1501–77) as writing that heather tea twice a day for 20 days would 'absolutely' break the stone.

Despite its classical heritage, however, heather has never been part of 'official' medicine. Perhaps its long association with areas of peasant poverty was against it?

Parkinson also noted the botanist Clusius (1526–1609) as claiming a heather flower oil helped cure 'the Wolfe in the face' or 'eating canker of the face'. This startling description could be an accurate word picture of the auto-immune disease lupus (the Latin for wolf).

Lupus is characterised, among many other symptoms, by a 'butterfly effect' of a rash that resembles bite marks. Where this becomes intriguing is in new evidence that heather protects for photosensitivity (see right).

Another Parkinson hint is that the distilled water can help dissolve tumours on the face – a potential marker for cancer research.

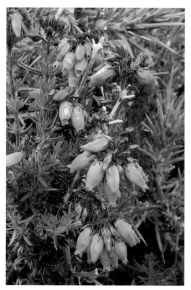

Modern research
2014 research confirmed the traditional antibacterial role of *Calluna vulgaris* tea or tincture in treating urinary tract infections. *E. coli* and *Proteus vulgaris* were controlled by the heather triterpinoids, including the newly named ursolic acid.

Similar findings emerged in 2013 for *Erica hebacea* (spring or snow heath) in neutralising *Proteus vulgaris*, a bacterium of the human intestinal tract. Earlier Scottish research (2010) had demonstrated that *Calluna vulgaris*, juniper and bog myrtle were all effective in treating the tuberculosis mycobacterium, again confirming old popular practice.

Most intriguingly, 2011 research indicated that *Calluna* is potentially photoprotective for the skin against UV rays.

Homemade heather ale
This is our own simplified recipe:

Take 28g (1oz) dried **heather tips** (we'd had ours in the airing cupboard for four months), and place in a large ceramic or glass bowl. Now add 200g (7oz) **local honey** (heather honey would be perfect) and 2 litres (3.5 pints) **warm water**. Sprinkle with ¼ teaspoon of **baker's yeast**.

Cover with a clean cloth, and leave in a warm place for a day or two until it starts to bubble. Strain into bottles and leave for another day to build up fizz, then refrigerate. Drink chilled.

It tastes 'yeasty' but refreshing, and will last up to a week if kept cold.

Heather ale
• refreshing
• nutritive

Heather tea
• cystitis
• prostate issues
• gout
• rheumatism

A fermented heather tea
Adapted from a modern Scottish recipe:

Pick **heather tips** and dry for at least a day. Liquidise to increase the surface area, and spread the mash onto a baking tray. Let it brew for three hours at room temperature. Then heat in the oven at 100°C until the contents are dry and crispy. Make as a tea on its own or mix with ordinary tea.

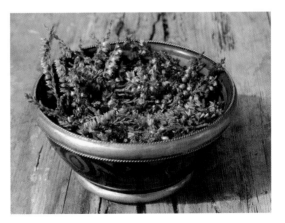

Herb robert *Geranium robertianum*

Herb robert is a familiar wild and garden plant that is almost too pretty to be called a weed. It has a rich folk history, with a perhaps surprising range of forgotten medicinal applications, which clinical research is now exploring and recovering.

**Geraniaceae
Cranesbill
(Geranium) family**

Description: Annual or biennial, to 50cm (20in); deep-cut delicate leaves with three or five leaflets; plant hairy, musky, often turning red; pink petals, round-edged, with white veins; stems form nodes at the base, turning red; shallow roots; seed heads have bulbous base and pointy tips, like a crane's bill.

Habitat: Edges of woods, hedgerows, gardens, walls, scree, shingle, waste land.

Distribution: Native in Eurasia, north Africa, North America; introduced to Australia.

Related species: At least 20 related cranesbills and hybrids; the closest botanically is the rare little robin (*G. purpureum*); shining cranesbill (*G. lucidum*) is commoner. American wild geranium (*G. maculatum*) has bluer flowers.

Parts used: Whole plant.

Herb robert is the commonest and among the best-loved of the European wild cranesbills or geraniums. Both family names refer to the beak-like appearance of the seed heads, as do the related storksbills (*Erodiums*).

Herb robert bears small bright pink flowers almost year-round in milder areas, and the attractive lacework of dark green leaves and pale moist stems with their characteristic nodes often turn bright red in summer and later.

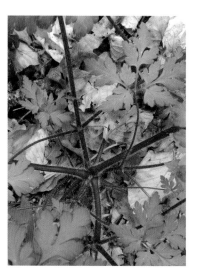

The redness is a key to the plant's place in folk memory and its long-held reputation as a herb connected to blood. The origin of the English name is elusive, and some commentators point to the Latin term *rubra*, for redness, as a possible source.

The first proper name associated with the plant is actually Rupert, probably St Rupert, a 7th-century Austrian bishop; a number of medieval, saintly Roberts, even a pope, have been linked with it, and then there is fairy tradition of 'robin' names (itself a diminutive of Robert).

Robin the bird, herb robert the plant and Robin Goodfellow – otherwise called Puck, the mischievous household sprite or hobgoblin – were intimately connected. In sympathetic magic their redness represented blood and life, but carried a darker meaning too, as a sign of ill luck or death: do not kill cock robin, do not uproot herb robert and do not cross Robin Goodfellow!

A multitude of common names for a plant suggests familiarity, affection, medicinal or foraging value, regional spread and long usage or wariness. The best British guide remains Geoffrey Grigson's pioneering book, *The Englishman's Flora* (1958). Grigson lists 110 British regional names for herb robert, and only one of these, death comes quickly, from Cumbria, refers to death as such. Nearly a quarter, 25 names, are variants on robert or robin; six are related to the plant's smell, and four to kissing. Most of the rest are descriptive rather than attributive.

Let us turn, then, to the matter of the plant's smell. The sweet-scented, large-flowered geraniums of the garden and house are actually Pelargoniums, hybridised from Southern African introductions in the seventeenth century. Pelargoniums are used in the perfumery industry and to make essential oils.

By contrast, crushed leaves of herb robert – one widespread name is stinking bob – have a musky smell that has been called disagreeable, foetid, mousy, foxy. John Pechey in 1707 was kinder: the smell was like parsnips, he thought.

Herb robert has hairs, but the scent is its main defence against predation. We can take advantage by crushing the leaves and rubbing them on the skin. This remains an effective repellent for midges and biting insects; maybe we should rename it 'herb rub it'! Crushing herb robert leaves

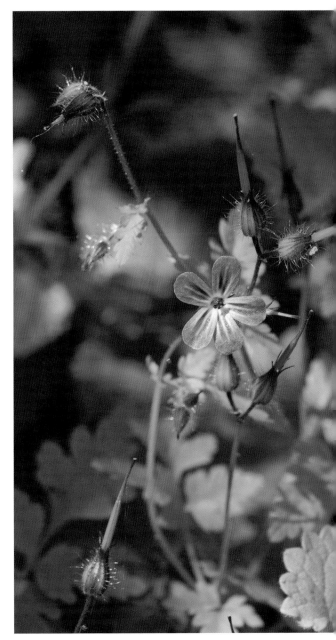

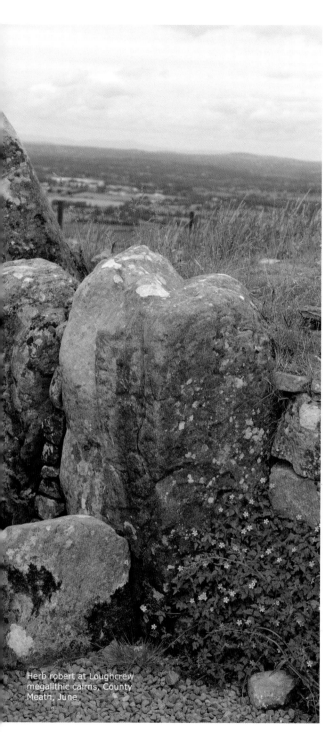

is an always available and easy medicine for gardeners, and it will also staunch everyday cuts.

Use herb robert for ...
Herb robert has a North American herbal counterpart, the wild geranium or alum root (*Geranium maculatum*), which is widely used and commercially available. Herb robert by contrast is now a largely forgotten herb, but has similar medicinal virtues.

These two geranium cousins are astringent, being high in tannins (*G. maculatum* has up to 30%), and vulnerary. As with other astringent plants, they have long been used for wound-healing and drying or clotting blood and other discharges.

In terms of blood-staunching, herb robert has been used in treatments for haemorrhage, metrorraghia, nosebleed, haemorrhoids and ulcers, especially peptic and gastric. In Ireland the plant was a favoured remedy for red-water fever, a disease of farm cattle.

'Other discharges' includes treatment for diarrhoea and dysentery, leucorrhoea, and excess breast milk and mucus.

In Southern Africa, a herb robert relative, *Geranium incanum*, is known as *Vrouebossie*, or woman's bush, and its tea is used in country areas to treat bladder infections, venereal diseases and menstruation-related ailments.

Herb robert at Loughcrew megalithic cairns, County Meath, June.

Another area of effective action of herb robert is for eruptions of the skin, including skin ulcers, tumours and eczema; Pechey in 1707 had already noted its value in treating erysipelas. A decoction of above-ground parts has been used as a mouthwash, for gum disease and for sore throat.

The kidneys are a site of traditional herb robert treatment, again in Ireland. The plant is mildly diuretic and cooling, and was used externally, in Ireland, for backache, eg as a compress soaked in herb robert tea.

Herb robert has juicy stems and is hard to dry – we found it resistant even to a dehydrator – so is most readily taken as a whole-plant fresh tea or tincture; the musky smell may not appeal to everybody, as we have seen.

A distilled water of herb robert has the same range of uses, as does a flower essence; its essential oil is worth consideration.

Finally, going back to the 'kissing' names, herb robert has a forgotten reputation as a mild aphrodisiac.

Modern research

Pharmacological research into herb robert is ongoing, and tends to confirm older uses. For example, work in 2010 found that a decoction of herb robert reduced blood sugar levels in rats with type 2 diabetes, supporting French folk tradition.

Herb robert has long had an underground reputation in treating cancers, especially of the skin, and tumours. Research (2004) into its high levels of the antioxidant germanium sesquioxide (organic germanium) supported such uses, but human clinical trials are still awaited and needed.

Additionally it has been shown that herb robert has antimicrobial potential, in treating *E. coli* infections (2012), and has been proposed as a possible AIDS treatment.

Finally, as an anti-inflammatory, an essential oil made from a combination of herb robert, clover and lavender proved effective in treating otitis, a painful ear inflammation (2014).

… though its scent is so disagreeable that the name of stinking crane's-bill is commonly applied to it, yet it is very pretty.
– Pratt (1866)

The herb bears closer investigation as a remedy. According to one authority it is also effective against stomach ulcers and inflammation of the uterus, and it holds out potential as a treatment for cancer.
– Chevallier (2016)

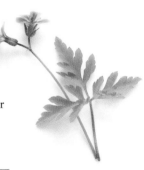

Harvesting herb robert
Herb robert is easy to harvest, but is so moist it is difficult to dry. We usually use it fresh. In mild areas the plant is available year round.

Herb robert tea
Put a sprig or two of **herb robert** per person in a teapot and cover with **boiling water**. Allow to steep for 5 or 10 minutes, then strain and drink, or allow to cool for use as a mouthwash or on the skin.

Herb robert tea
• mouthwash
• wash cuts & grazes
• antioxidant
• drink after X-rays
• drink after dental work

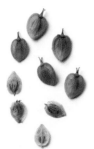

Hogweed *Heracleum sphondylium*

**Apiaceae
(Umbelliferae)
Carrot family**

Description: A common tall wayside plant flowering from summer into winter. Hairy stem and leaves.

Habitat: Waysides, damp meadows, waste ground, field margins.

Distribution: Throughout the British Isles, common in Europe across to Asia. Introduced to North America.

Related species: Giant hogweed (*H. mantegazzianum*), the other species found in Britain, mainly near rivers, is phototoxic. Cow parsnip (*H. maximum*) and other species are used in North America very much like hogweed.

Parts used: Young shoots, flower buds, roots and seeds are eaten and used as medicine.

Warning: Do not confuse with giant hogweed, *H. mantegazzianum*, which can grow to 3m tall and causes severe skin damage in sunlight.

Hogweed's abundance tends to obscure its virtues. Foragers prize its delicious celery-like shoots, farmers have long fed it to stock (yes, including pigs), and herbalists of old valued it, particularly Native Americans using the related cow parsnip.

Hogweed has been described as the *commonest tall wayside white umbellifer of the* [British] *summer and autumn*. The North American equivalent, the cow parsnip (*Heracleum maximum*), is equally well distributed, a common sight along highways, in fields and on waste lots.

The vigour of the Heracleum genus is honoured by reference

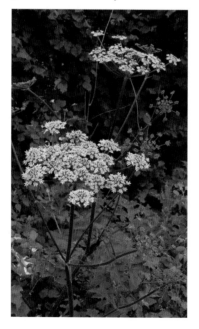

to the hero Heracles (in Greek) or Hercules (Latin). The common name hogweed is a little less heroic, reflecting the old use of the plant for feeding pigs and other livestock. As a modern forager points out, the flowers also smell foetid, which is rather 'unglamorous' to humans but appealing to insect pollinators.

Hogweed shoots, buds and seeds (both green and brown when mature) are favourites with foragers, and are enjoyed in traditional Baltic food and drinks culture. Hogweed also has long-established – if forgotten – herbal uses and potential new ones.

But there's another side we should address first, that of identification. Many people associate the word hogweed with the closely related giant hogweed (*Heracleum mantegazzianum*), a huge and impressive plant that can soar to 3 metres (14 feet) in a growing season. It prefers riverbanks, and is luckily much less widespread than its edible cousin.

It is wrong to say, as is sometimes seen, that giant hogweed is

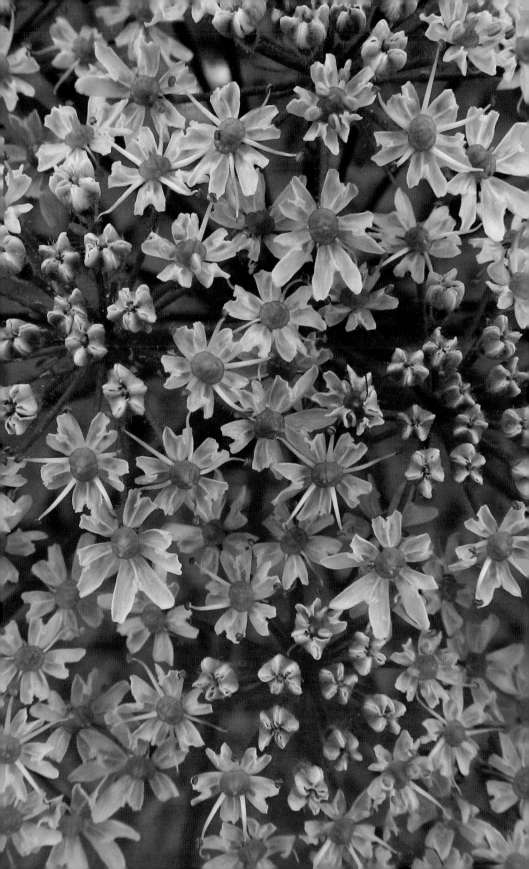

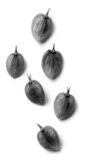

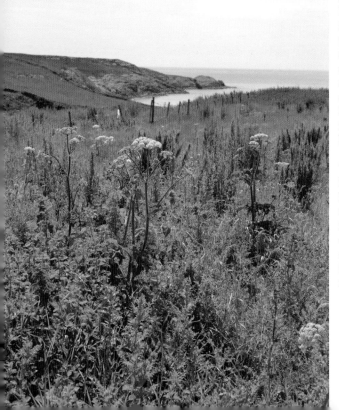

Hogweed above the cliffs, Anglesey, June

poisonous, but it is phototoxic. As its defence mechanism against predators the plant secretes furanocoumarins in its sap and bristly hairs. In the presence of sunlight these phytochemicals can cause contact dermatitis, with severe blistering and possible long-term purpling of the skin.

In hot sunny weather, hogweed can have a similar but much less severe phototoxic potential. If weeding or strimming hogweed, do wear gloves. Strimming shreds the stems and scatters the sap far and wide, so goggles too are a good precaution. Watch for your children picking hogweed stems for making blowpipes or toy boats, especially in the hot sun, and keep them away from giant hogweed.

Use hogweed for...
In North America cow parsnip was one of the most used Native American and First Peoples' wild herbs, as was hogweed in pre-revolutionary Russia and the Baltic states.

The medicinal range of both herbs was administered by root decoctions or tinctures. In North America cow parsnip root tea eased colic, cramps, headaches, colds, flu and tuberculosis, while poultices externally went on sores, bruises, stiff joints and active boils. In European herbalism Linnaeus knew hogweed as a sedative in 18th-century Sweden, while two centuries earlier in England Gerard advised it for headache and lethargy; in the mid-17th century Culpeper proposed it for epilepsy and jaundice. In modern French herbalism hogweed root is a male aphrodisiac and for high blood pressure (hypertension).

The European experience is interesting since it encompasses both stimulant and sedative roles for hogweed. The inference is that it works at neurological level, depending on dose and patient constitution, as an amphoteric, ie capable of opposite actions, or normalising function.

Contemporary American herbalist Matthew Wood draws attention (in discussing cow parsnip) to the work of the late William LeSassier, who found that chewing some seeds of *Heracleum* was 'revelatory', heightened sensitivity and conferred psychic benefits. We found the green seeds of hogweed to have a similar effect. This area suggests a line of further research, as do the older traditional uses.

Modern research
Research in 2008 identified novel uses for the Heracleum genus as an anti-asthmatic, and for memory and 'alertness-improving' effects.

Hogweed was used (2013) in tests of rat thoracic aorta to produce the first evidence for its vasorelaxant properties, supporting traditional anti-hypertensive therapies. Octyl butyrate, a component of the essential oil of hogweed, was shown (2014) to be cytotoxic to certain human melanoma and carcinoma cells.

Webster et al (2010) isolated anti-mycobacterial constituents in cow parsnip root, including several furanocoumarins, supporting former use for treating infectious diseases, specifically tuberculosis.

In addition to anti-fungal and anti-mycobacterial properties, the root of cow parsnip (2006) demonstrated antiviral actions, by means of immunostimulation.

This study demonstrates that aqueous extracts of the roots of H. maximum [cow parsnip] ... possess strong in vitro antimycobacterial activity, validates traditional knowledge, and provides potential for the development of urgently needed novel antituberculous therapeutics.
– Webster et al (2010)

Harvesting hogweed
Hogweed provides several harvests through the year. The young **leaf shoots** are picked in the spring, and have a pleasant taste. Our favourite wild vegetable is the **flower buds**, picked while they are plump but still encased by the leaf base, making a neat little packet for steaming. The **seeds** can be nibbled green, when they have a strong smell of mandarin orange, or gathered when they mature and turn brown, then having a more complex spicy citrus flavour. **Roots** are best harvested from young plants in the autumn or the following spring.

[Hogweed shoots are] ... unequivocally one of the best vegetables I have eaten.
– Phillips (1983)

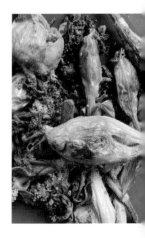

Hogweed flower buds
Lightly steam **hogweed flower buds**, then fry them gently with **butter** and **garlic**.

Well-being tea
Per cup of boiling water, use a teaspoon of **green hogweed seed** and a couple of leaves of **ground ivy**. Cover and leave to infuse for 10 or 15 minutes, then strain and drink.

We find this tea clears the head and relaxes the body. It makes a good evening tea.

Lesser celandine *Ranunculus ficaria* syn. *Ficaria verna*

Once you identify lesser celandine correctly (it's not greater celandine and not figwort), you have an effective, old but also modern remedy for the painful condition of haemorrhoids. External use of the plant is safe, but it is potentially toxic if taken internally – not that this discourages braver foragers, who appreciate the young leaves.

**Ranunculaceae
Buttercup family**

Description: To 30cm (12in) tall, with rosettes of long-stalked, glossy and heart-shaped leaves, usually with paler inner markings; bright star-like yellow petals, 7–12, often 8 in number, with three green sepals; both fibrous and whitish tuberous roots.

Habitat: Damp woodland, waysides, gardens; invasive, often forms massed colonies.

Distribution: Abundant in Great Britain, except for north Scotland and parts of Ireland; throughout Europe, temperate Asia; introduced to North America.

Related species: Several subspecies, some of which spread by seed and others by bulbils; these subspecies can be used interchangeably for medicine.

Parts used: Whole plant, especially the tubers.

One of the earliest spring plants is the lesser celandine. It has such a pleasing combination of stars and hearts: the flowers are star-like, golden, almost shiny-enamelled; and the leaves are glossy green, heart-shaped, low to the ground.

By looks it should be, and is, of the buttercup (Ranunculus) family, but it is the only species of 600 or so with a safe external herbal use. In general, buttercups are acrid and toxic, causing blistering of the mouth and gastro-intestinal tract in cattle and humans alike, and are best avoided.

In Britain lesser celandine grows in colonies, forming swathes of yellow in damp woodland, by ditches and in gardens from February to May. Coming from winter gloom, you need all the light you can get, and this plant is a pleasure to behold.

In some areas of the northern USA and Canada, though, the proliferation of introduced lesser celandine is an alien invasion, swamping native plants like trilliums. It holds its own against ground elder in our own garden!

Poets and novelists have been engaged, entranced by this early brightness. Wordsworth preferred it even to his beloved daffodils. It was a shame, then, that Wordsworth's memorial in Grasmere has the wrong celandine, the sculptor repeating a common confusion with the unrelated greater celandine, but this time permanently in stone.

DH Lawrence had his character Paul Morrel in *Sons and Lovers* describe lesser celandine as *scalloped splashes of gold, on the side of the ditch*. Like Wordsworth, Lawrence enjoyed the way the flowers open and close with light, and *press themselves against the sun*.

Anonymous country-dwellers also joined in the fun: among names recorded for it are butterchops, crazy bet, cups, gentleman's cap and frills, golden guineas, spring messenger and starlight.

But all this spring profusion relies on what is underground, a root system that has fibrous roots and attached small tubers – *a broom handle festooned with potatoes*, as one modern writer calls it.

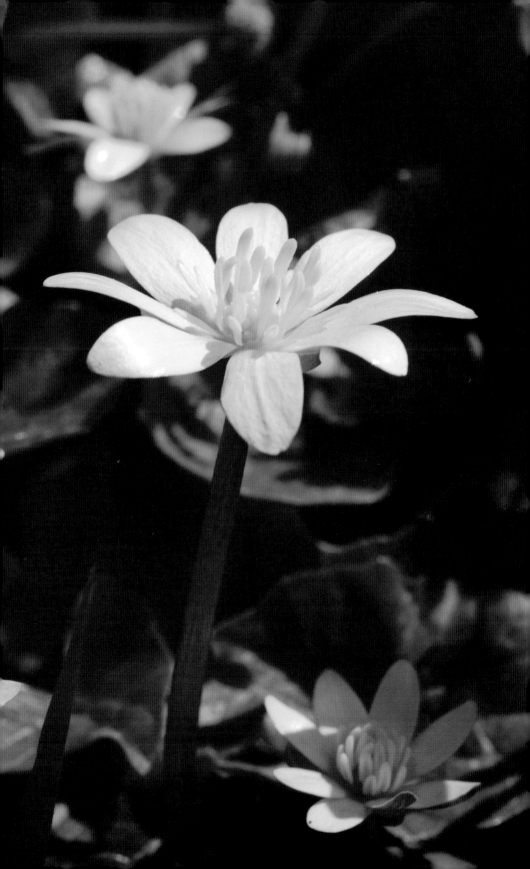

Use lesser celandine for ...

Each tuber is a storehouse from which a new plant emerges, and the tubers are the medicinal part, gathered in spring or autumn.

These white tubers were the 'figs' that gave rise to the plant's generic name *Ficaria*; another old European name, again confusingly, is figwort (the true figwort is *Scrophularia nodosa*). In the USA lesser celandine is also called a fig buttercup.

At one time, notably in Germany, the earliest-appearing leaves of lesser celandine were collected, as a remedy for scurvy. They do contain high levels of vitamin C, but also become toxic as the season progresses, owing to rising amounts of protoanemonin.

On the other hand, some contemporary foragers regard the leaves as safe and, with cautions, recommend them in stir fries and, in small amounts, in wild salads. The cooked tubers resemble potatoes in taste; these are recorded as a survival food in parts of Scotland.

But everyone knows the tubers for another reason. They are also termed 'piles' for their resemblance to haemorrhoids, and the plant is still called pilewort.

Haemorrhoids are a painful condition of dilated veins and swollen, protruding tissue at the anus. The piles can be internal or external. The condition often occurs in pregnancy or after childbirth.

Lesser celandine is an effective treatment, with its saponins soothing the inflamed tissue and its tannins toning the veins. A decoction is made into an ointment or a hot compress.

Nicholas Culpeper, in 1653, went further: it worked *by only carrying it about one, (but if he wil not, bruise it and apply it to the grief)*. In other words, merely carrying the plant in some form would do, but if needed, apply it to the piles.

The medicine was and remains effective, but was it found by trial and error or by 'design', in that the plant's appearance gave a clue, a 'signature' for its ordained human purpose? Was lesser celandine a confirmation of the now long-discredited doctrine of signatures?

The modern consensus is that effect probably preceded cause; in the words of one commentary, *As in other cases, however, this may well be merely a post-hoc rationalisation*. Parkinson (1640) agrees that usage came first: *it is certaine by good experience*. The salient fact is that lesser celandine genuinely works in treating haemorrhoids.

It was also used to treat scrofula, or King's evil, a tubercular complaint of swollen glands in the neck, and for lumps and corns (the true figwort has similar uses).

Modern research

There are no contra-indications for external use of lesser celandine, though a case report (2015) found that a 36-year-old woman suffered acute hepatitis after 'consuming' lesser celandine for haemorrhoids. Other factors such as alcohol or drug over-use were eliminated in this case. However, it seems she had been taking the plant internally as a tea, which is not a typical modern treatment regime for the plant.

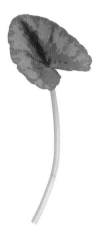

Other haemorrhoid herbs

Anti-inflammatory (demulcent) and astringent (tannin-rich) herbs can be used in addition to or to replace lesser celandine in piles treatment. Rose family astringents, eg avens and agrimony, have been found effective, as are marigold, witch hazel (*Hamamelis virginiana*), horse chestnut or oak, in ointment or distilled water form.

Note that these are *topical* piles treatments. The *cause* of the piles, probably poor digestion and constipation, or liver dysfunction, should be addressed simultaneously; fibre, say, should be introduced to the diet gradually.

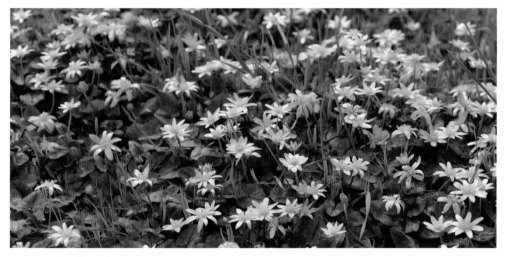

Lesser celandine ointment

Gather lesser celandine in early spring when they are in flower. If you are weeding them out of your garden, dig up the whole plant including the small tubers, but if you are harvesting wild plants you can just use the leaves and flowers.

Lesser celandine ointment
• haemorrhoids
• varicose veins

Cover the **lesser celandine** with **olive oil** in a saucepan. Simmer gently for about 20 minutes, then strain out the plant material and return the oil to the pan after measuring it. For every 100ml of oil, add 10g **beeswax** or 5g candelilla wax. Stir on low heat until the wax has melted. Pour into jars and leave to set before putting lids on and labelling.

Mouse-ear hawkweed *Pilosella officinarum*

Asteraceae
Daisy family

Description: Low-growing perennial, to 30cm (12in); *for detailed description, see adjacent text.*

Habitat: Drier short grassland and rough meadows, also rocky areas, sand dunes.

Distribution: Native to Europe and Western Asia; naturalised in USA and Canada, but an alien in some states and provinces; a notifiable noxious weed in Australia and New Zealand.

Related species: Other Pilosellas include shaggy mouse-ear hawkweed (*Pilosella peleteriana*); tall mouse-ear hawkweed (*P. praealta*); fox and cubs (*P. aurantiaca*); yellow fox and cubs (*P. caespitosa*). Each of these have subspecies, and hybridisation is frequent.

Parts used: Above-ground parts, as tea, tincture, juice, distillation.

Mouse-ear hawkweed is a useful but neglected herb, with specific actions for treating whooping cough and brucellosis. As these painful conditions have declined in the West, so has its own reputation. But it retains powerful antibiotic properties for home treatment of coughs, colds, bleeding, diarrhoea and fevers.

In early summer the bright yellow single flowerheads of the diminutive mouse-ear hawkweed twinkling by a ditch or on rocky soil are a pleasure to the eye, with forgotten medicinal benefits.

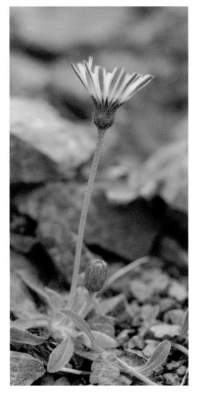

Sir John Hill in 1812 praised mouse-ear hawkweed as *an exceedingly pretty plant* [with] *scarce any smell but an austere bitterish taste.* He was outdone by Leo Hartley Grindon in 1859 (right).

Botanically, mouse-ear hawkweed occupies its own genus, the Pilosella, classified between the hawk's beards (Crepis) and the hawkweeds (Hieracium) of the Aster tribe. Until recently, it was called a Hieracium, specifically *Hieracium pilosella.*

It can all get very baffling, but the plant itself, fortunately, has clear distinguishing marks.

William Curtis's idealised portrait of the plant opposite shows the characteristic creeping stolons or runners, the cropped layers of sulphur-yellow florets on a single longish stem, the paddle-shaped and hairy 'mouse' ears in rosette leaves (green above and whitish below), and the alternating orange-red stripes under the calyx, like a medieval jousting tent.

The under-surface redness is an interesting feature of mouse-ear hawkweed, with its closest Pilosella relative being the russet-flowered fox and cubs (*P. aurantiaca*). There are other Pilosellas, listed left, plus various hybrids, which share medicinal properties with it.

It is worth clarifying that the plants known as *mouse-ears*, aka mouse-ear chickweeds, are unrelated members of the Cerastium genus, in the pinks or Caryophyllaceae family. We use the full English name mouse-ear hawkweed to avoid confusion.

We won't go into the further historical complications of the plants named *Myosotis* (Latin for mouse ear), which became the forget-me-nots (now in the Borage family) – John Parkinson in 1640 classified the blue forget-me-not alongside mouse-ear hawkweed as *Myosotis scorpioides repens*, the 'small creeping blew Mouseare'.

Use mouse-ear hawkweed for …
Mouse-ear hawkweed has a long history in treating respiratory disorders by soothing coughs, colds, asthma and bronchitis.

It is a herbal specific for whooping cough, a highly infectious disease generally treated by vaccination in developed countries. Epidemics still occur, and treatment is long and not always successful.

Mouse-ear hawkweed can be used alone in herbal whooping cough treatment or combined with other

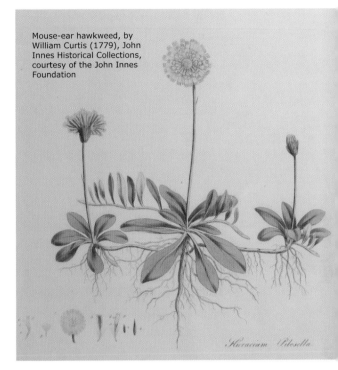

Mouse-ear hawkweed, by William Curtis (1779), John Innes Historical Collections, courtesy of the John Innes Foundation

recognised 'antitussives' such as mullein and coltsfoot.

The *British Herbal Pharmacopoeia* of 1983 gave a whooping cough mixture using mouse-ear hawkweed, white horehound, mullein and coltsfoot, although this recommendation had been dropped by the 1996 edition.

Mouse-ear hawkweed can be called a stimulating expectorant, which works by loosening stubborn phlegm and helps in ejecting it by increased salivation. It is also astringent and partly diuretic, which explains its action

It has been received into the [apothecary] *shops under the name of* Auricula muris, *and considered as possessing an astringent quality; but at present, in this respect, is but little regarded.*
– Curtis (1779)

[It grows in] *dry hedgebanks, delighting in the most sunny and drouthy conditions, where it can bask in the noontide ray … *[the blossoms]* in favourable seasons, and when in perfection, have the smell of raspberry jam.*
– Grindon (1859)

in toning inflamed muscle and in treating diarrhoea.

It was once a familiar wound herb, with its astringency also found useful in treating excessive menstruation or haemorrhaging. It was recommended for nosebleeds and piles, an action supported by its known antibiotic qualities.

Mouse-ear hawkweed is regarded as specific for treating brucellosis, a bacterial infection caught by people from infected livestock or milk. This presents as intermittent (sometimes called undulant or Malta) fever, which has been largely controlled worldwide.

Medicinally, the bitterish stem sap is swallowed or the plant boiled

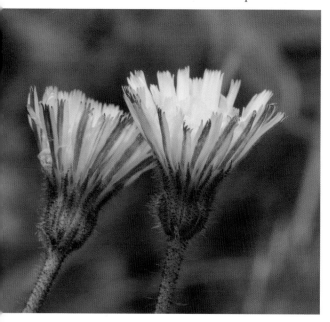

fresh as a decoction. A distilled water can be made, for either drinking or external application – used, as Pechey wrote, for *wound-drinks, Plaisters and Ointments*. Hill suggested boiling the leaves in milk for external use.

Some herbalists believe the fresh herb is more effective than the dried. Indeed, Julian Barker (2001) suggests a reason for the plant's fluctuating reception over time is the weak action of the dried form.

At one time mouse-ear hawkweed had a reputation for improving the eyesight, but this was based on a persistent belief that hawks (Greek *Hierax*, which gave the name Hieracium) would swallow the bitter sap to sharpen their own keen vision. Falconers were also said to feed their birds a tea made from mouse-ear hawkweed.

While a benign plant in its native Europe, mouse-ear hawkweed is condemned as an alien weed in some states and provinces of the USA and Canada, New Zealand, Australia and Japan. It can form impenetrable mats that crowd out native grasses grazed by stock. New South Wales's government, for example, classifies all hawkweeds as class 1 noxious weeds, which citizens must report for eradication; Hawkweed Alert is the online interactive program.

Modern research
A European Union herbal monograph on mouse-ear

hawkweed (2015) limits itself (citing lack of data) to use of tea or powder for urinary tract disorders.

Polish research meanwhile (2011) has identified a new isoetin derivative, a flavone, that was a strong antimicrobial, which reduced colon carcinoma cell line proliferation.

The Haudenosaunee people of New York state (2010 research) use yarrow and mouse-ear hawkweed, among other plants, as antimicrobials for treating diarrhoeal and stomach ailments, notably for forms of salmonella poisoning.

Serbian research (eg 2009), has confirmed mouse-ear hawkweed is high in umbelliferone, an antibiotic coumarin responsible for the anti-brucellosis action of the plant. Umbelliferone absorbs UV light, and has an application in sunscreen products.

Mouse-ear hawkweed relaxes the muscles of the bronchial tubes, stimulates the cough reflex and reduces the production of catarrh. This combination of actions makes the herb effective against all manner of respiratory problems, including asthma and wheeziness, whooping cough, bronchitis and other chronic and congested coughs.
– Chevallier (2016)

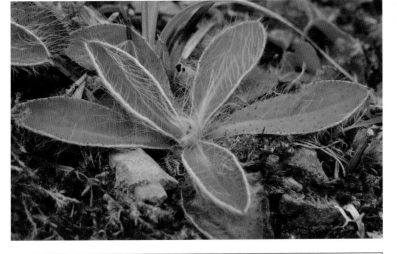

Identifying mouse-ear hawkweed: left, basal rosette; opposite, close-up of flowers

---

Syrup of mouse-ear hawkweed

Harvest when **mouse-ear hawkweed** is in flower. Put your pickings in a pan, cover with **water** and boil. Simmer gently for a few minutes, remove from heat. Cover pan, and leave overnight to infuse.

Strain off the liquid and pour into a clean pan. Add 200g sugar for every 250ml of liquid. Bring to the boil, stirring until sugar dissolves. Warm receiving bottles, pour syrup in, add cap and label.

Dosage: 1 teaspoonful 3, 4 or more times a day, according to need.

Syrup of mouse-ear hawkweed
- specific for whooping cough
- catarrh
- congested cough
- disorders of urinary tract

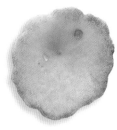

Navelwort *Umbilicus rupestris*

Navelwort is a common and attractive, almost alien-looking presence in shady West Country lanes and woodland edges, but its medicinal properties, as reflected in its various 'wort' names and ability to cool inflammation, are unduly overlooked.

Crassulaceae
Stonecrop family

Description: A fleshy native perennial bearing spikes of greenish white bell-shaped flowers in summer. The stalk attaches to the centre of each leaf, leaving a dimple or navel on the top.

Habitat: Hedgebanks & stone walls in high rainfall areas.

Distribution: Fairly widespread in Ireland, and found primarily in the western parts of Britain.

Similar species: Marsh pennywort (*Hydrocotyle vulgaris*) has a similar leaf but is in the pennywort family.

Parts used: Leaves.

A member of the stonecrop family of British succulents, navelwort or wall pennywort is a distinctive plant growing in colonies on sheltered walls, hedgebanks and tree roots, mainly in the west of the British Isles.

On paper at least, it might be confused with several other navelworts in unrelated families: blue-eyed mary or navelwort (*Omphalodes verna*) is a garden plant of the borage family; the marsh pennywort (*Hydrocotyle vulgaris*) of the pennywort family grows in wetlands and has pink flowers; and gotu kola (*Centella asiatica*), also called the Asiatic pennywort and Indian water navelwort, is an important Ayurvedic herb.

The English names of navelwort suggest an enduring popular esteem: a plant does not earn 'wort' status without proving itself medicinally (or for brewing). It has been known as navelwort since medieval times for the way its central dimple in the leaf resembles a belly button (it is named *umbilicus* in Latin). Another 'wort' name hinting at function,

current in both John Parkinson (1640) and Maud Grieve (1931), was kidneywort.

The name pennywort is a reference to the greenish-grey of the fleshy, round leaves, which look like an old silver penny; it has also been called moneypenny, penny cake, penny leaves and similar coin-related names.

Other common names hint at its herbal uses or virtues: it was cut-finger (wound-healing), corn leaves (applied to corns or warts) and coolers (probably for its value in relieving the pain of burns).

In classical terms, navelwort was *Umbilicus veneris*, the navel of Venus, to the Romans, and still to Parkinson. The name was not, however, matched by an equivalent aphrodisiac reputation, despite efforts by William Coles, in *The Art of Simpling* (1656).

If its names have been colourful and expressive, navelwort's distribution has been surprisingly stable, in always having a western bias in the British Isles. It was probably more widespread in

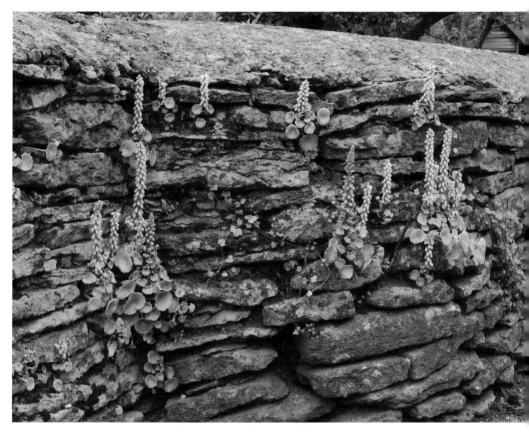

pre-industrial times – Parkinson said 'it groweth very plentifully in many places of this kingdome'.

As if to hint at the plant's gradually reduced distribution, the first edition of Gerard's *Herball* (1597) describes a navelwort plant growing on stonework in Westminster Abbey near to Chaucer's grave. The second edition, by Thomas Johnson (1633), omits this reference, no doubt because the plant had gone.

Use navelwort for ...
Navelwort was once accepted in 'official' medicine: in Culpeper's English version (1653) of the *Pharmacopoeia Londinensis*, the reference book for physicians and apothecaries, it was recommended for 'kib'd heels [kibes were ulcerated chilblains], being bathed in it, and a leaf laid over the sore'.

It had been excluded from similar lists by the nineteenth century. Nonetheless it was once a

Navelwort on a wall in Gloucestershire, June

significant herbal presence, and it could be turned to much more by today's herbalists and first aiders.

It is the leaves that are used, for their watery, cooling sap – it is a close relative of the houseleek (*Sempervivum tectorum*), sometimes called the English *Aloe vera*, which has similar soothing uses.

The herbalist Julian Barker describes pulping navelwort leaves with a rolling pin and applying the mash to tired or sore eyes, to piles and chilblains. Using a compress or poultice will prolong the contact time.

Parkinson provides the most complete herbal perspective. The leaves, either in extracted juice or distilled water form, he

[The flower spike looks] *like an upright fibre-optic wand with miniature bulb lanterns all the way up it.*
– Raven (2011)

Among the most interesting-looking leaves you are likely to put on a plate.
– Irving (2009)

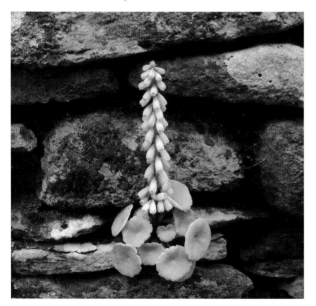

tells us, are 'very effectuall for all inflammations and unnatural heates'. He describes some of these: inwardly for 'a fainting hot stomacke' or hot liver, the bowels or womb; and outwardly, for pimples, redness, St Anthony's fire (the skin condition erysipelas), and for sore kidneys.

Navelwort leaves are also used to break stones in the kidney and liver, he says, to relieve 'wringing paines of the bowels and the bloody flux [dysentery]', and are 'singular good for the painefull piles or hemorroidall veines'.

Parkinson recommends an ointment, either of navelwort leaves alone or mixed with myrrh, for easing painful 'hot goute, the Sciatica and the inflammations and swellings of the cods [testicles]'. The plant is partly diuretic, and could relieve 'dropsie' (water retention or oedema), and would reduce 'the Kernells or knots of the neck and throate called the Kings Evill' (scrofula).

Navelwort was good for emergencies with 'greene' (fresh) wounds and burns: the skin of the leaves was removed, he said, and the juice or an ointment from it rubbed on the wound. The skin itself made a ready plaster for a splinter, and when left in place for a day or two would draw it out.

Parkinson does not advise the use of navelwort to treat epilepsy, which Mrs Grieve reported as an 'old reputation'; she said the practice was revived in the 19th century but added that the plant had no permanent reputation as an epilepsy remedy. The last reference to navelwort being considered for petit mal concerned flower essence developer Dr Edward Bach, who from 1930 to 1932 experimented with it as a flower remedy, but dropped it.

Navelwort leaves are edible, though John Pechey in 1707 was unenthusiastic: *The Leaves are fat, thick and round, and full of Juice, and taste clammy.* Contemporary foragers have proposed them for salads, stir fries and sandwiches.

Modern research
A 2012 ethnobotanical study found *Umbilicus rupestris* being used by a diaspora Slavic community in south-central Italy. They crushed the leaves, mixed in pork fat and soot, and put them on foruncles (infected hair follicles).

Showing there is nothing new under the sun, this is very close to a recipe in the Anglo Saxon *Old English Herbarium*, dating to about the year 1000, for *Cotyledon umbilicus*, the same plant. In this recipe equal quantities of the plant and pig's grease (the recipe specified using 'unsalted' grease for women) were pounded together and placed on a swelling, which would soon disappear.

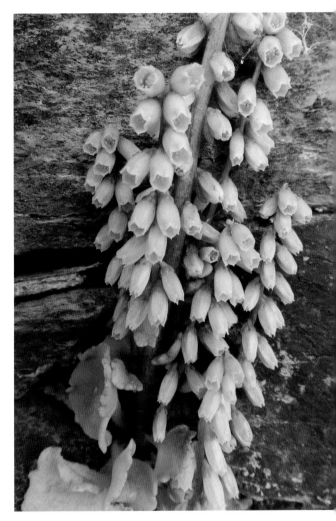

Fresh poultice
Use the fresh leaf as a poultice for burns and minor injuries as well as placing on hot swellings such as boils. Simply split the leaf and apply the wet side to the skin, or crush and apply, holding in place with a sticking plaster.

Fresh poultice
- burns
- boils
- haemorrhoids
- splinters
- cuts
- pimples

Ox-eye daisy *Leucanthemum vulgare*

Ox-eye daisy is a larger relative of the humble common daisy, and shares many of its medicinal virtues. In both cases modern herbalism has overlooked what these plants can offer, and the time might be right for a reconsideration.

**Asteraceae
Daisy family**

Description: A bright, sprawling meadow perennial of high summer, whose flowers consist of a large golden central disk, surrounded by numerous long white ray petals. Flowers borne on open, branching stems to 1m (3ft) high, flopping over as they age; short, stubby dark green leaves; roots shallow.

Habitat: Grassland, gardens, road verges, waysides, especially on rich soils.

Distribution: Across whole of British Isles but less common in Scottish Highlands; native in Europe, Middle East, north Africa; introduced to North America, Australasia.

Related species: A medium size between the much smaller native common daisy (*Bellis perennis*) and the larger Shasta daisy (*Leucanthemum x superbum*), sometimes a garden escape.

Parts used: Leaves, flowers.

The name 'daisy' derives from the Anglo-Saxon 'day's eye', from the way the flowers open up as the sun rises. Unlike the familiar common or lawn daisy, ox-eye daisy, its larger relative, stays open at night too, being almost luminescent in moonlight, and much the brightest plant presence on summer evenings.

This was noticed long ago – one of ox-eye's old names is moonflower. So here is a plant of both sun and moon, as its flowers symbolically indicate. The original scientific name given by Linnaeus in 1753, *Chrysanthemum leucanthemum*, ie 'gold flower, white flower', perfectly and euphoniously captured the plant's duality.

What a pity, then, that the current name, corrected in the 1990s, in Latin means only 'common white flower' – though in referencing ox-eye's abundance science is reflecting the problems ox-eye is posing for farmers, as we will see.

It is indicative of popular affection for a plant when it has a variety of common names, indicating local variations in appearance or

use over time. Geoffrey Grigson's wonderful *The Englishman's Flora* (1958) certainly gives a long list for ox-eye daisy.

Among the regional names he notes are billy button, butter daisy, cow's eyes, devil's daisy, dog daisy, dundle daisy, fair maids of France, gools, grandmothers, horse blob, horse daisy, maudlin, midsummer daisy, mother daisy, open star, povertyweed, rising sun and white gowlan.

Another name for ox-eye is marguerite, long a familiar garden flower. It is said to be named for Margaret of Anjou, the French wife of King Henry VI. Strictly, though, marguerite is the large white daisy from the Canary Islands, *Argyranthemum frutescens*.

Its popular names do carry hints of a shadow side to ox-eye, as in 'devil's daisy'. What can be welcome in the garden might be anathema to the farmer.

Ox-eye growing unchallenged in a field could indicate that the land was being neglected, and in England Henry VI introduced

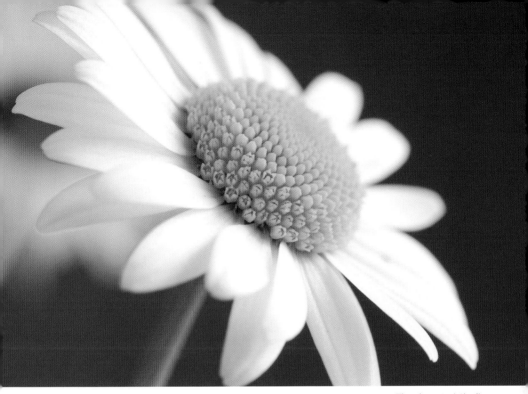

punishments for aberrant farmers. In medieval Scotland the presence of 'gools' in grassland led to fines of one wether [castrated] sheep.

In modern Australia there are records of their ox-eye daisies causing contact dermatitis in some people, and you find similar warnings in websites from the American West. Indeed, this beloved wild and garden flower in Europe is seen as a destructive alien weed in hotter, drier climates (purple loosestrife and St John's wort are among other examples).

What happens is that the plant's own protective mechanisms are exacerbated in more extreme conditions. Ox-eye stems develop a bitter, acrid juice that makes the plants unpalatable to grazing cows and pigs, as well as insects and most human foragers.

A close relative of the ox-eye is *Chrysanthemum cinerariifolium* – quite a mouthful in Latin, but better known in English as pyrethrum, the most effective natural insecticide – and ox-eye shares some of its qualities.

The website for Colorado State University highlights that ox-eye has no natural biological controls, that cows won't eat it and insects keep away from it. This leads to ox-eye pushing out other plants that stock animals prefer to eat.

In hot, dry conditions it only takes five days for the plant to set viable seed, which can lie dormant in the ground for some years. The plant has a shallow root system, as European gardeners know, but once the seeds are in the ground, it will come back again and again, no matter how often it is uprooted.

The characteristic disc (yellow) and ray florets (white) of ox-eye daisy

Flowers [of the Greater Wild White Daisie] *cast forth Beams of Brightness.*
– Pechey (1707)

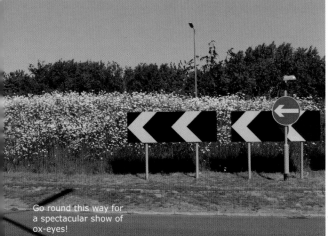

Go round this way for a spectacular show of ox-eyes!

Externally, ox-eye tea has an ancient reputation in lotion or compress form to relieve wounds and bruises; in Ireland it was used to bathe sore eyes. In these conditions its medicinal range is similar to that of chamomile, another distant relative.

Salmon (1710) advocates ox-eye distilled water for ruptures of the bowels and as a vehicle for other medicines. Likewise he maintains that its liquid juice heals any inward wound, spitting of blood and ruptures: take with *a glass of old Malaga or Red Port Wine*.

It consolidates and conglutinates the Lips of Wounds to a Miracle.
– Salmon (1710)

The fresh leaves chewed, have a sweetish, but unpleasant and slightly aromatic taste, somewhat like parsley, but not hot or biting; they have been recommended in disorders of the breast, both asthmatic and phthisical, and as diuretics, but are now seldom called for.
– Green (1820)

Use ox-eye daisy for…

Records of modern herbal use are sparse, which can lead to both 'bioprospecting' of older texts and also practical experimentation at a time when the plant is spreading. A herb does not lose medicinal power when it goes out of fashion – it is still there, particularly in wild strains, and available to try out for yourself.

The herbals suggest that ox-eye has a history as an antispasmodic, especially for whooping cough and asthma. It is tonic and sweat-inducing, the boiled root being effective in reducing night sweats.

The flowers made into an infusion are recorded as helping relieve chronic coughs and bronchial distress. Sir John Hill's *Family Herbal* of 1812 mentions that the 'great daisy' is 'balsamic and strengthening' for the lungs.

We found making an ox-eye flower essence to be wonderful. One recent year, early June marked Julie's birthday, a full moon and a lunar eclipse all at the same time. Julie began her moon essence at sunset, around 9 pm, and left it overnight from moonrise to moonset. Then on the summer solstice she made an all-day ox-eye sun essence. Both were profound in their effect, but markedly differing: the moon essence was predictably cooling and calming, the sun essence warming and stimulating.

Modern research

Research has been sparse and focused on the plant's physiology, speciation and cases of contact dermatitis, but a 2015 report found the plant had potential in crude oil phytoremediation, surviving exposure to the oil and enhancing reduction of crude oil in soil.

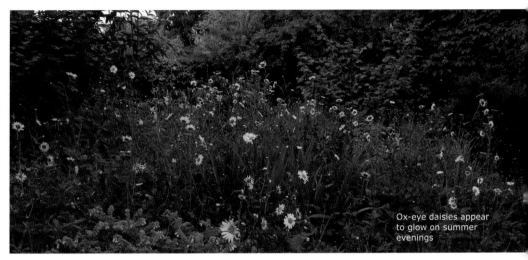

Ox-eye daisies appear to glow on summer evenings

Ox-eye daisy oil

Pick **ox-eye daisies** on a dry day. Spread out on a cloth or some paper and allow them to dry for a day or two, then fill a jar with them. Pour in **extra virgin olive oil** to fill the jar, stirring to release any air bubbles. Cover the jar with a piece of cloth or gauze held in place with a rubber band or string. This allows any moisture to escape. Leave in a warm sunny place for a few weeks.

Strain off the oil, which will have a peculiar daisy smell, into a bottle and label. You can add a few drops of essential oil to perfume the oil if you wish – choose oils that enhance the therapeutic use of the oil, such as eucalyptus, lavender or chamomile. Use as a chest rub for stubborn coughs, or on muscles for bruising or aches and pains.

Ox-eye daisy oil
- chest rub
- difficult coughs
- bruises
- aching muscles

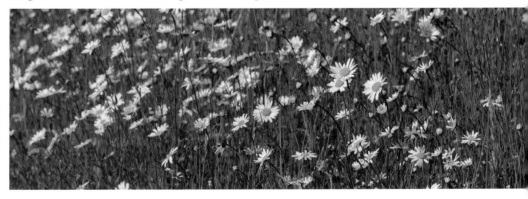

Scots pine, Herefordshire,
May

Pine *Pinus* spp.

Pine has multiple human uses, providing pitch, tar, timber, kernels, sap and resin. It is a specific for respiratory issues, a disinfectant and antiviral.

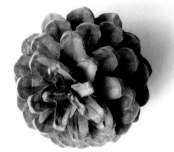

Pinaceae
Pine family

Description: (Scots pine) height varies with soil, wind and other conditions, from dwarf to 30m and more (100ft); takes irregular pyramidal shapes, often with broken branches; fissured red-brown bark near the crown, greyer below; thin needles in pairs, grey-green; buds sticky with resin; male flowers yellow, female pink; cones green, grey-brown to brown.

Habitat: Scots pine are native only in small areas of the Caledonian Forest, but much planted in woods, heaths, shingle throughout Britain.

Distribution: The family is largely forest trees of the cool/cold temperate north; Scots pine is native to northern Europe; in North America by 1600.

Related species: The conifers include firs, spruces, larches and cedars as well as pines; the only other British native conifers are the threatened juniper (*Juniperus communis*) and yew (*Taxus baccata*). Some 100 pine species worldwide have similar uses.

Parts used: Bark, needles, resin, distilled water, tar.

Scots pine, also known as Scotch pine (or fir), is a conifer (cone-bearing) evergreen tree that has similar uses to other pines, but is one of only three British native conifers, with juniper and yew.

Pine has multiple uses, much like the date palm or coconut in their own cultures. It was prized first as a timber, for ships' masts, pit props, telephone poles and railway sleepers; in the First World War pine forests were felled for ammunition boxes and trenching.

The tree itself gives tar and turpentine, used in paints and varnishes, and a volatile oil for cosmetics and perfumes. Pine resin went into glues used in boat-building and for sealing wax and, when ground into powder, as rosin for violin bows.

Pine pitch was the oil of pine, widely used as an antiseptic and a preservative: amber, or fossilised pine resin, preserves insects from as long ago as 125 million years. In Traditional Chinese Medicine amber is called *hu po*, and was once used in urinary tract infection and for stones.

Although native Scots pine disappeared from most of Britain some 5,000 years ago through climatic warming, stumps and branches were preserved in many peat bogs. These pine remnants were resinous and provided free fuel and (unreliable) lighting until the early 19th century when oil lamps became popular.

Pine sap produces a potent wine; the roots could be used for ropes, and the cones give a brown dye. The 16th-century herbalist Pietro Andrea Matthiolus noted that distilled green 'apples' (cones) yielded a face wash much used to remove wrinkles.

At about the same time as Matthiolus, the first Spanish travellers to North America saw that inner bark of pine was a survival food of the native Americans; Linnaeus also describes it, mixed with flour, for a similar purpose in the Sweden of his time (mid-18th century).

More palatable of course are the silky-smooth pine kernels, which have long been a basis of Mediterranean food, including in Pharaonic Egypt. Parkinson in 1629 noted their various use by *Apothecaries, Comfit-makers, and Cookes*. He said medicines made from pine kernels were *good to lenifie* [soothe] *the pipes and passages of the lungs and throat, when it is hoarse.*

Parkinson added the 17th-century truism that pine kernels *stir up bodily lust and encrease sperme*. We offer a recipe mixing pine nuts into an electuary with liquorice and cardamom to test his words.

That pine kernels are reputed to be aphrodisiac seems appropriate for a tree once sacred to Artemis, the moon goddess who presided over childbirth. The pine cone was a symbol of virility. This isn't all myth: our culture still chooses pine trees for Christmas celebrations and the yule log.

The scent of pine is distinctive – refreshing, clean, masculine (or so the advertisers want us to believe). It has been thought therapeutic in itself, and this belief underlay the siting of tuberculosis sanitaria within the pine woods of the Swiss Alps in the 20th century.

The scent is disinfectant, as we all know from commercial air fresheners that use pine scent. But this isn't new: Parkinson in 1640 wrote of *our ordinary Francumsence* [pine resin] *that is usually burned in houses and chambers, to aire and perfume them.*

Pine steam inhalations are a specific treatment for respiratory problems, using the bark or essential oil, along with drinking pine needle tea. Pine essential oil can be added to hot baths. Herbalist Peter Conway recommends 10 drops of pine oil with 5 ml of almond oil (carrier) poured into a hot bath as it fills; he says it is *wonderfully penetrating and relaxing, helping to release muscular tension.*

The famous Vicks Vaporub was originally made from cedarleaf and turpentine oils, among other ingredients. Patented in the US in 1894, it is now called Vicks and manufactured from petroleum-based products. It is well known for easing bronchial congestion, but any form of pine rub or massage oil will actually have similar value.

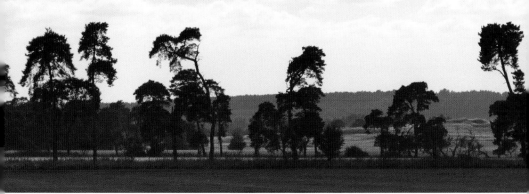

The sound of pines, as the wind eases through their tops, is comforting. The lovely old words soughing and susurrating are onomatopoeic efforts to capture this quality, while Keats said *pines shall murmur in the wind*.

So, pine is a tree that both smells and sounds special. It was also planted in special places – British examples include on warrior graves in Scotland, as landmarks along old droving routes and along beaches, and to form a row of windbreaks in the Norfolk and Suffolk flatlands.

All the same, as writer Charlotte du Cann argues, most conifers in Britain *stand unrespected in suburban parks and plantations*, whereas in America, in *a citadel of conifers*, in her words, the pine remains *a wild and ancestral tree, a world tree that grows in forests of great power and resonance*.

But modern research may be changing this picture, with pine gaining reputation as a 'functional food', that is, a medicinal food, and its traditional herbal uses being scientifically authenticated.

Use Scots pine for...
Not surprisingly, pine has a particular affinity for the respiratory system for conditions ranging from coughs to tuberculosis, strep throat and asthma. It is excellent in both early and late stages of colds to eliminate mucus (expectoration) and control infection.

Ireland-based herbalist Nikki Darrell points out that pine is particularly valuable for treating asthmatics who have been on long-term steroids. Steroids have been connected with adrenal insufficiency, and pine acts as an adrenal restorative.

The late American herbalist Michael Moore has a useful ascending scale for pine actions.

He rates a tea of pine needles as pleasant-tasting, mildly diuretic and expectorant. The inner bark used as a tea and sweetened with honey is stronger, and valuable in the later stages of a chest cold. Pine pitch, the size of a currant, chewed and swallowed, makes for stronger expectoration again, with the softening of deep mucus.

Backround scene: planted rows of Scots pine, near Mildenhall, Suffolk, October

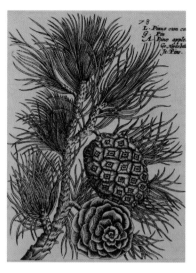

*Pine Needle Tea, made
by pouring 1 pint of
boiling water over
about 1 ounce of fresh
white pine needles
chopped fine, is about
the most palatable pine
product I have tasted.
With a squeeze of
lemon and a little sugar
it is almost enjoyable.*
– Gibbons (1966)

Another American herbalist,
Matthew Wood, characterises
pine as a stimulating antiseptic.
It is used externally in the form
of baths, poultices (for sores and
burns) and for direct placement on
wounds.

Native Americans are among
many pine-based cultures to find
that pine sap will prevent wound
putrefaction, and help eliminate
splinters and even bullets.

Pine's stimulating/antiseptic
qualities extend further into
proven efficacy for promoting
blood circulation, as a laxative
and an astringent, for relieving
colic and headache, for soothing
rheumatism, arthritis and oedema,
and as an aphrodisiac. Finally,
Pycnogenol is a commercially
made extract from the bark of
Pinus pinaster.

Modern research

Pine contains a category of
flavonols called oligomeric
proanthocyanidins (OPCs).
These serve to protect the body's
collagen against cell damage
and thereby have a role in cancer
prevention; moreover OPCs
have been shown to slow the
accumulation of fat in the arteries
and reduce risks of heart disease.

Hence pine may have a supportive
role in counteracting two of the
major life-threatening conditions.
What else is research showing?

More initials for one thing!
Research on mice (2009a) indicates
that pine's polyphenyl propanoid-
polysaccharides complex (PPCs)
inhibit allergic IgE reactions,
notably in asthma. Asthma
treatment costs $8 billion annually
in the US.

Pine has been shown (2005a) to
be more effective than resveratrol
in inhibiting growth of yeast
infections *Candida albans* and
Saccharomyces cerevisiae. It is also
effective against the bacteria
Staphylococcus aureus (2000).

Drug-makers are taking note
of these potentials, including
Pycnogenol, in an extract of
French maritime pine bark (2002),
as also the possible role of pine as
a 'functional food', namely one
that contains bioactive compounds
that have been shown to help
relieve chronic health problems
(2005b, 2009b).

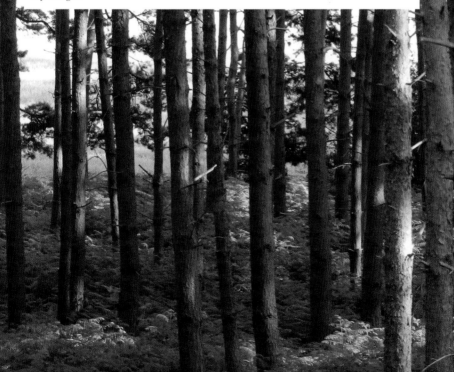

Pine needle tea

Use a small bunch of **pine needles** per cup of **boiling water** in a teapot. Steep for 10 minutes, then strain and drink. Can also be used as a steam inhalation. The dried needles have a more soothing, soapy feel. Add honey or sugar to your taste.

Pine needle hydrolat

Place a steep-sided bowl upside down in a large stockpot. Place **pine needles** around the upside-down bowl, then pour in enough **water** to cover the needles – it should not be deeper than the bowl. Place another bowl on the first one, right side up. Put the lid on the stock pot upside down, so that it is lower in the centre. Gently heat until the water starts to boil. Put ice on the upturned lid to help condense the steam that is collecting. The steam will condense and drip down into your bowl, making your hydrolat (aromatic water).

Passionate pine electuary

Grind together in a food processor: 3 tbsp **pine nuts**, 3 tbsp **dates or raisins**, 3 tbsp runny **honey**, 1 tbsp **liquorice powder**, 1 teasp **cardamom powder**. This is a version of an old love potion; take a teaspoonful several times daily for relieving dry coughs.

Primrose & cowslip

Primrose, *Primula vulgaris* & Cowslip, *Primula veris*

These bright spring flowers cheer the spirits after long, dark winters, and are among Britain's favourite wild plants. They were once important medicinals, but could well be used again as safe remedies for treating insomnia, migraine, catarrh, arthritis and rheumatism, among other historic uses.

Primulaceae
Primrose family

Description: Perennials with large crinkly green leaves and pale yellow flowers in spring.

Habitat: Old woodland, ditches, hedgerows, banks, grassland and churchyards. Cowslips prefer more open grassy areas.

Distribution: Primrose is widespread through the British Isles, cowslips less common in north and west. Native to Europe and temperate Asia. Cowslip introduced to north-eastern US.

Related species: Oxlip (*P. elatior*) is a separate, rare species. The hybrid of primrose and cowslip is known as false oxlip, *P. x polyantha*. Bird's eye primrose (*P. farinosa*) and Scots primrose (*P. scotica*) have violet or purple flowers and a localised distribution.

Parts used: Roots, flowers, leaves.

Cowslip is an under-used but valuable plant. – Chevallier (2016)

Primroses are one of the earliest spring wild blossoms – the name comes from 'prima rosa' or first flower (*primavera* in Spain and Italy). They are often still blooming when the taller cowslips join them a few weeks later.

It is the spring flowers that people love most. A survey carried out by the charity Plantlife in 2015 showed that bluebells were the nation's most popular flower, with primrose second and cowslip fifth. Perhaps it is their colour and freshness charming us after the long, dark winter, and no doubt these are the plants we loved in childhood, with early memories of woods and meadows.

Primrose attracted approving names, such as darling of April and ladies of the spring. But cowslip was from Old English 'cow-slop', or a plant springing up where cows in meadows deposited their dung.

If that was rather down to earth, cowslip was also known as bunch of keys or St Peter's keys, a name inspired by the hanging flowers. These resembled the bunch of keys that St Peter metaphorically carried and could open the kingdom of heaven to a believer.

Interestingly, this name was a deliberate Christianising takeover of an earlier pagan (Norse) name: cowslip was once dedicated to the goddess Freya, the virgin of the keys. The keyflower plant or cowslip would open her own sexual kingdom. Such a myth had to be reconfigured!

The nodding head of cowslip may also have suggested a palsy (paralysis), and other ancient names included palsywort, paralytica and arthritica, the latter for the use of the roots for rheumatic and arthritic pain relief.

Coming up to date, cowslip has made a gratifying dramatic recovery from centuries of overpicking for making the popular cowslip wine or syrup. This practice has fallen into decline, and meanwhile local councils have widely planted cowslip on British roadsides as part of a meadow mix, ensuring that highways and waysides are an opportunistic new habitat for this much-loved flower.

Use primrose and cowslips for…
Primrose and cowslips have similar medicinal properties, though cowslips are more often used and have a deeper healing profile.

One abiding reputation of cowslip has been as a 'nervine', a plant that benefited the nervous system, in this case as a relaxing sedative. Hildegard of Bingen (1098–1179) was among the earliest European commentators on cowslip, which she recommended for melancholia, in the form of a compress of tea made from the plant, held over the heart while sleeping – in modern terms, an antidepressant remedy.

Both plants have been used to treat insomnia. Austrian naturopath Maria Treben (1982) met a man

… to ease paines in the head [primrose and cowslip are] *accounted next to Betony* [Stachys officinalis], *the best for that purpose. Experience likewise hath shewed, that they are profitable* [effective] *both for the Palsie, and paines of the ioynts, … which hath caused the names of* Arthritica, Paralysis, *and* Paralytica *to bee giuen them.*
  – Parkinson (1629)

A basket of primrose and cowslip flowers

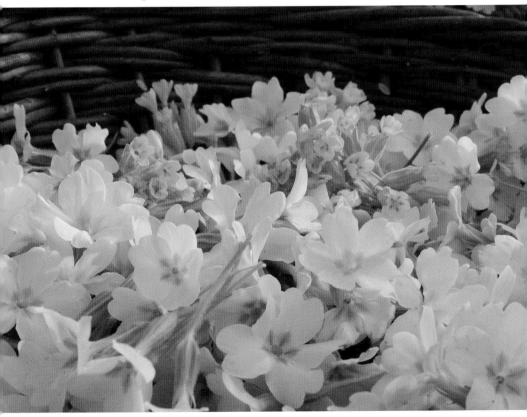

The Water of the Flowers, the Conserve, and the Syrup [of cowslips] are Anodine, and gently provoke Sleep; and are very proper Medicines for weakly People.
– Pechey (1707)

The flowery May [hawthorn], who from her green lap throws, / The yellow cowslip and the pale primrose.
– Milton (1632)

who could not sleep despite taking strong sleeping pills. Her remedy for him was a tea of dried plants: 10 parts cowslip, 5 of lavender, 2 St John's wort, 3 hops and 1 valerian root. A powerful mixture, it cured his sleeplessness within a week.

Cowslip wine was a well-liked method of adding a sedative effect to the pleasant alcoholic buzz, and it was extended to pacifying unruly children, if the Tulliver children in George Eliot's novel *Mill on the Floss* (1860) are drawn true to life.

The plants' profile also includes relief of headaches and migraines, panic attacks and nervous tension in general. Pechey in 1707 approved eating cowslip flowers and leaves as potherbs and in 'sallets': they were 'very Agreeable to the Head and Nerves'. They remain good to eat. Pechey also noted cowslip as anodyne, or pain-relieving, which science confirms through its salicylate content.

Cowslip has an antispasmodic quality too, with its saponin-rich roots proving to be strongly

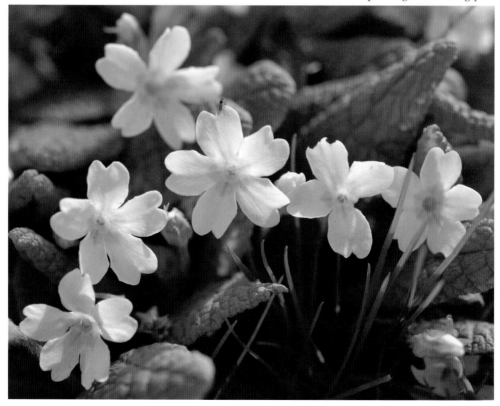

expectorant. A decoction of cowslip roots was once a familiar remedy for clearing phlegm and congestion, whooping cough and bronchitis. It is 'official' in Germany for catarrh, and may well have an unexplored value in asthma treatments.

In terms of 'palsy', as mentioned, one former use of the plants was to treat vertigo or loss of balance. John Wesley's herbal (1753) suggested for this: ... *drink Morning and Evening, half a Pint of Decoction of Primrose-root.* The other older uses for arthritis and rheumatism are explained by the salicylates in the roots having anti-inflammatory properties.

Cowslip also has a diaphoretic or sweat-inducing quality that underlies its fever-breaking and detoxifying potential.

It is a safe remedy for babies, children and the old. The flower essence-maker Saskia Marjoram sums up her experience of the flower as offering *a safe mothered feeling that enables you to skip with joy.* Avoid both plants, however, if you have a known intolerance to aspirin or salicylates.

Modern research
Polish research (2012) indicated the mechanism of the flavone zapotin as a chemopreventive and chemotherapeutic (anti-cancer) agent. First named in 2007, zapotin is extracted from the leaves of *Primula veris* (cowslip).

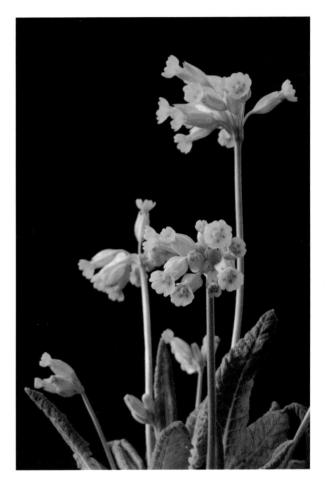

Placebo-controlled, randomised double-blind trials (1994) into the German-made tablet, Sinupret, confirmed its decongestant effect in acute sinusitis. Sinupret contains extracts of *Sambucus nigra* (elder) flowers; *Primula veris* (cowslip) flowers; *Rumex acetosa* (sorrel) plant; *Verbena officinalis* (vervain) plant; and *Gentiana lutea* (gentian) root.

Cowslips (above) and primroses (left) by a country lane in Norfolk

Caution: Avoid taking cowsip and primrose if you have a known aspirin allergy or salicylates intolerance.

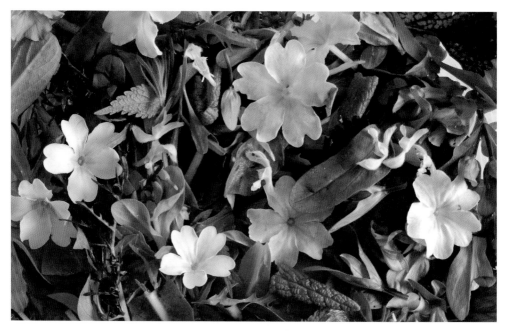

Primrose flowers and young leaves are a pretty addition to spring salads

Harvesting primroses and cowslips

Primroses flower for several months in the spring, with cowslips starting a little later. Only pick wild primroses and cowslips where they are plentiful. Garden varieties of primula can also be used.

Primrose or cowslip tea

Pick a few **primrose and/or cowslip flowers** per cup of **boiling water**. Infuse for about 5 minutes for a lovely golden, soothing cup of tea.

Primrose tea
- coughs
- anxiety
- insomnia
- colic

Primrose conserve
- dry coughs
- sore throats
- insomnia
- colic

Primrose or cowslip conserve

Fill a small jar with **primose and/or cowslip flowers**. Pour in **runny honey**, stirring to remove any air bubbles. Leave in a warm place for a few weeks, until the flowers have faded.

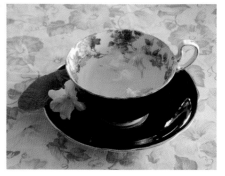

Strain out the spent blossoms. Take a teaspoonful for sore throats or digestive upsets.

Purple loosestrife *Lythrum salicaria*

Purple loosestrife is the old water-loving 'long purples' but is also called a 'purple plague' in parts of the USA where it is seen as an unwanted invader. Remarkably, it has a toxin-leaching role in land-healing or phytoremediation that is paralleled in a range of traditional and novel medicinal applications.

Purple loosestrife is a striking and glamorous British wild plant whose tall magenta flowerheads add delight to summer wetlands or wayside ditches. Gardeners too have taken to it – one notes how *its reliable drama has led many of us to grow it in damp spots in our gardens.*

Purple loosestrife stands tall and strong, as the old country name 'long purples' suggests. Its vigour can also be problematic for humans. In Fenland dykes it was once known as 'iron hard' for its impenetrable root system, which broke farm workers' shovels. It has become 'purple plague', the 'poster plant' of invasives in parts of the US.

Lythrum is thought to be from a Greek term for blood because the plant has an old medicinal reputation as a blood stauncher.

Salicaria is 'willow-like', for the plant's thin, tapering leaves; it was once called purple willowherb. Salmon (1710) hedges his bets: he says the name was given *because it grows among willows, or … has willow-like leaves.*

And 'loosestrife' itself? Refer to an old herbal, such as Salmon's, and you will find the yellow and purple loosestrifes described together in the same genus, the *Lysimachia*. It was only in the later 20th century that the two plants

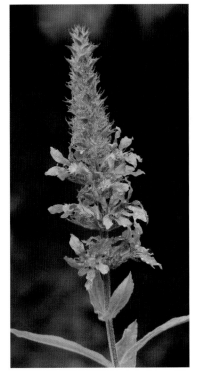

Lythraceae
Purple loosestrife family

Description: A highly attractive perennial and vigorous coloniser, to 1.5m tall (5ft), with many erect, angular stems; bright magenta-purple flowers, whorled, with typically 6 floppy petals; leaves narrow, lance-shaped, untoothed; deep taproot and lateral roots.

Habitat: Forms colonies in watersides, whether wetlands, fens, ponds, rivers or ditches; can persist when soils dry out.

Distribution: Native to Europe, but also SE Asia and east/south coasts of Australia; naturalised in North America, and considered invasive in east, midwest and far west.

Related species: Perhaps surprisingly, not the yellow loosestrife (*Lysimachia vulgaris*), which is a Primula; the water purslane (*Lythrum portula*) is the closest relative, along with the rare grass poly (*L. hyssopifolium*).

Parts used: Above-ground parts.

were separated, with the yellow reassigned to the Primulaceae (but keeping the name *Lysimachia vulgaris*) and the purple given its own genus, *Lythrum*.

Lysimachus was a fabled king of ancient Sicily, and his name consists of two elements meaning 'undo' and 'war' – or 'loose strife'.

He is said to have been the first to use the plants to calm tetchy oxen in ploughing teams. When placed under the yoke, resting on the oxen's shoulders, the plant deterred the biting insects that abound in marshy areas. The oxen were duly pacified and their 'strife' brought to an end.

Names can only take us so far, of course, but early European colonists in North America seem to have used the plant to good effect with their own fractious oxen, and both forms of loosestrife made smudge sticks or incense to keep insects away from humans.

The first record of the plant in North America was in 1814, in an eastern port, following a presumed accidental introduction via a cargo of ballast from Europe. Lacking soil and plant predators of its native habitat, the plant prospered, spreading through river systems west and north, becoming larger and massier as it did so, reaching Alaska by 2001.

The charge is that it overshadows and outperforms native wetland plants, such as the bulrush-like cattail (*Typha latifolia*), and creates impenetrable colonies or disturbs irrigation channels. Purple loosestrife is well equipped to be a coloniser, with one plant putting up 30 to 50 stems and, in a recent calculation, some 2.7 million tiny seeds a year. Unavailing clearance efforts are said to cost upwards of $45 million annually in the US.

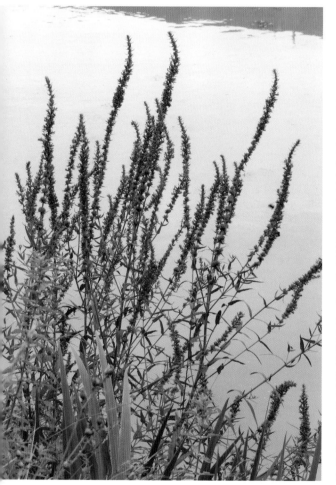

But American herbalists, notably Timothy Lee Scott and Jim Mcdonald, have raised counter-arguments to the conservation orthodoxy. They say purple loosestrife can work to rehabilitate wetlands by absorbing excess nitrogen and phosphorus from fertiliser and pesticide runoff.

In fact, the plant has remarkable powers of phytoremediation or land-healing, Mcdonald notes. That is, like other so-called 'green liver' plants, purple loosestrife can neutralise chemical contaminants such as lead or the banned polychlorinated biphenyls (PCBs).

Use purple loosestrife for …
Purple loosestrife is astringent and tannin-rich enough to have been used to tan leather, but its astringency is mitigated by a high mucilage content that eases inflamed tissue as it tones it.

This unusual combination of properties underlies the plant's reputation in both Western and Chinese medicine for treating diarrhoea, dysentery ('bloody flux'), leaky gut, irritable bowel and many forms of discharge with blood and inflammation. It was found effective in the 19th century for use in epidemics of infant cholera and typhus, and its role in treating epidemic infection is as yet under-researched.

The plant was a wound herb, and John Parkinson among other herbalists recommended an ointment made with butter, wax and sugar for 'wounds and thrusts'. Another aspect of purple loosestrife's affinity for blood discharges is its historic role in treating excessive menstrual bleeding, via a vaginal douche.

The distilled water, Parkinson wrote, *likewise clenseth and healeth all foul ulcers and sores wheresoever, and stayeth their inflammations, by washing them*. The water, he added, was also effective as a gargle for painful inflammations like quinsy (throat abscess) and the king's evil (scrofula, a tubercular swelling of the lymph nodes). Applied externally, it also helped remove spots and scars, such as those from smallpox and measles.

Parkinson also noted that *the distilled water is a present remedy for hurts and blowes on the eyes, and for blindnesse*, provided the vitreous humour was not damaged.

Parkinson's biographer, Anna Parkinson (a probable descendant), had a remarkable confirmation of this assertion. She told us she once had something painful in her eye, and remembered what Parkinson had written about purple loosestrife.

She didn't panic, but calmly made a water distillation of the plant. When it was ready, she applied the liquid to her eye, which gave ready relief – this seems to us a courageous example of faith in a mentor!

Purple Loosestrife offers great potential as a valuable and practically useful medicinal, possessing an admirable balance of astringent and mucilaginous properties.
– Mcdonald (2013)

[The liquid juice is] *of an exceeding binding Quality … Dioscorides says it is good to stay all manner of Bleedings at Mouth or Nose, or of Wounds, or any other Bleeding whatseover. … [It stops] all fluxes of the Belly, even the Bloody-flux [dysentery] it self.*
– Salmon (1710)

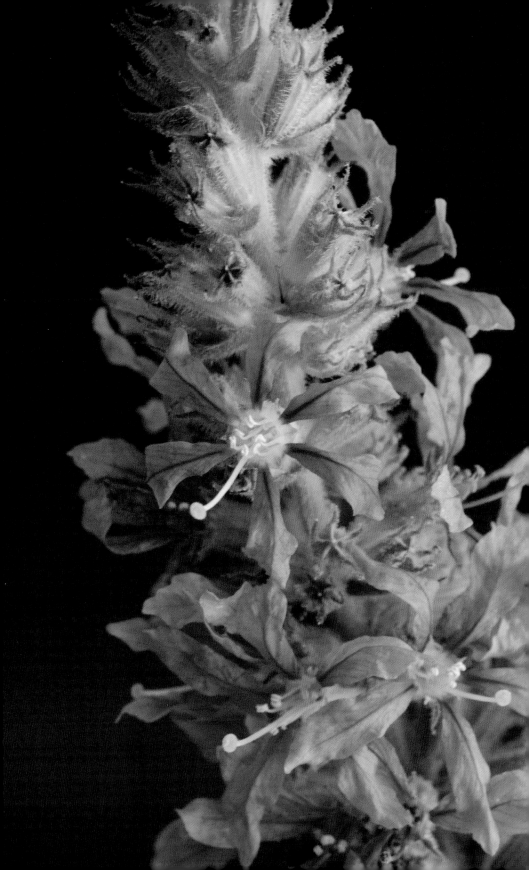

Purple loosestrife is 'superior' to eyebright in preserving the sight, said Mrs Grieve, and Timothy Lee Scott points out that it offers a widely available alternative to this plant, which has been over-harvested in the wild in the US.

The distilled water can also be used as a poultice for drying/toning any painful external condition, and is safe for children.

Another area of growing interest in purple loosestrife's actions is as a powerful antibacterial, antifungal and antimicrobial.

Modern research

Writing in 1931, Mrs Grieve commented that purple loosestrife is *Scarcely used at present medicinally, but once esteemed.* Things have changed, and there is now a growing body of recent research that has identified some of the active principles of purple loosestrife's wide range of pharmacological actions.

Work by a European team (2010) showed that *in vitro* purple loosestrife has 12 types of glycoconjugates; three of these showed complete inhibition of plasma clot formation, but two others were pro-coagulant. This suggests that, like yarrow, purple loosestrife is amphoteric with respect to blood flow, that is, it can act both as a coagulant (the traditional use) and an anti-coagulant at different times.

The plant's glycoconjugates were also demonstrated (2012) as having greater antitussive and bronchodilatory effects than the drug salbutamol.

The anti-inflammatory properties of purple loosestrife were shown (2015) to result from tannins identified as ellagitannins, and specifically dimeric salicarinins.

Earlier research (2005) supported purple loosestrife's effectiveness against the pathogenic fungus *Cladosporium cucumerinum* and the bacteria *Staphylococcus aureus*. The ester vescalagin was isolated as the active principle of the antibacterial activity. Purple loosestrife is definitely a plant worth using.

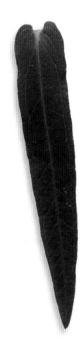

Purple loosestrife ointment

- fungal infections
- bacterial infections
- cuts & grazes
- blemishes

Purple loosestrife tea

- loose bowels
- fungal infections
- bacterial infections
- cuts & grazes
- blemishes

A quick purple loosestrife ointment

Pick **purple loosestrife** while in flower, or leaves whenever available. Chop up and cook gently in enough **ghee** (clarified butter) or **coconut oil** to cover for about 15 minutes, then strain out the plant parts and pour into clean jars. Note that coconut oil will be liquid in hot weather.

Purple loosestrife tea

Put a sprig of **purple loosestrife** per person in a teapot, and cover with boiling water. Steep for 5 to 10 minutes. Strain and drink, or cool for external use on the skin or as an eyewash.

Rowan *Sorbus aucuparia*

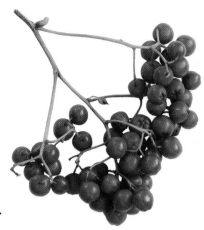

A handsome tree through the seasons, rowan is far more than a city ornamental. The name rowan stands for protection, and it was used across northern Europe as a charm against witchcraft for livestock, homes and the individual. Herbally a rose family astringent, it is made into a tea and tincture, the famed jelly and an ancient form of ale.

Rosaceae
Rose family

Description: A small deciduous tree, growing to 15m (50ft); slender and elegant in form: silvery-grey trunk in winter, bright green pinnate, ash-like leaves in spring, frothy white flowers in summer and bright orange-red berries in autumn.

Habitat: Woodland, wayside, mountain and marginal land; grows at higher altitudes than any other native British tree.

Distribution: Northern and western parts of British Isles; native to temperate Asia, Europe; naturalised in North America.

Related species: Whitebeam (*Sorbus aria*), wild service tree (*S. torminalis*), the American mountain ash (*S. americana*).

Parts used: Berries, bark.

Rowan's common names attest to its ancient importance as a tree evocative of fresh life (quicken, wicken or wiggen, quickbeam) and magic (witchbane, witchwand, witchbeam). It is both enchanting to behold and protects against enchantment.

More prosaic is its descriptive name mountain ash (often used in North America). True, it thrives on poor mountain soil, but it is no ash, merely having ash-like leaves.

The Latin species name *aucuparia* hints at rowan's attractiveness to birds in the autumn and winter, when migrant fieldfares, redwings and waxwings descend on berry-rich British rowan trees, gobble the fruit and spread the seeds. An *auceps* was a fowler, who used rowan's berries as a lure; hence an old name, fowler's service tree.

'Rowan' itself, as befits a plant whose association with man goes back to prehistory, has various suggested origins: a Norse word similar to 'rune', protection; a

Swedish term for redness; or a reference to a spinning wheel, for which rowan wood was often used. The genus name *Sorbus* is for the service trees and beams.

A beautiful and compact tree, rowan is beloved of civic planters as a quick-growing ornamental for roadsides, parks and churchyards. This is the tamed version, though, and rowan remains at heart a wild pioneer tree, growing in dwarf forms at higher elevations and latitudes, fighting for a foothold in inclement weather, and coping with browsing deer or sheep, or moose in Scandinavia.

Protection is the keyword for rowan's role, for stock and homes as much as people. But carrying pieces of rowan loose or wrapped in red twine as charms has never appealed to authority. Take the book *Demonologie* (1598) where King James VI of Scotland (and I of England) condemned *such kinde of Charmes as commonlie dafte wives uses … by knitting roun-trees … to the haire or tailes of the goodes.*

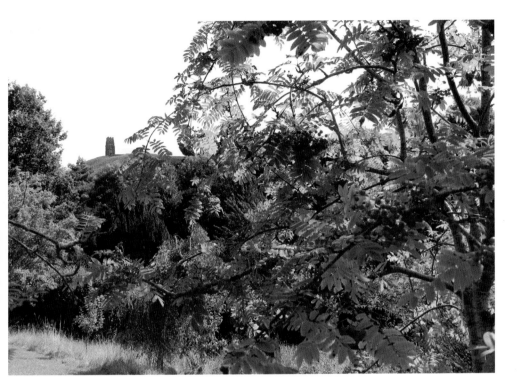

Use rowan for ...

Rowan is a rose family astringent, and the bark is tannin-rich. It is a traditional tea or tincture for treating diarrhoea, piles, vaginal discharge and menstrual pain. The bark is also a dye (black and orange) and once used in tanning.

The fruit is nutritive, if tart. It has only a little pectin, which is why crab apple is added in making the famous jelly to help it set. A decoction of the berries with added apple and sugar is a country remedy for whooping cough. A rowan gargle is used for sore throats. Its diuretic quality helps in strangury (inability to urinate), and it is used for rheumatism and arthritis. It is a useful anti-inflammatory for sore kidneys.

Cooking rowan alters its irritant parasorbic acid to the more tolerable sorbic acid, which underlies the general advice to avoid taking it in raw forms.

Modern research

The service tree (*Sorbus domestica*) inhibits aldose reductase, which may be useful in diabetic complications (2008), and the related *Sorbus commixta* has potent anti-inflammatory effects (2010).

Fruiting rowan in the Chalice Well garden, under Glastonbury Tor, August

Their spells were vain. The hags return'd To the Queen in sorrowful mood, Crying that witches have no power, Where there is Rown-Tree wood.

– The Laidly Worm of Spindleston Heugh, *a tale of a Northumberland dragon (13th century or earlier)*

Rowan jelly
- digestive upsets
- diarrhoea

Rowan syrup
- coughs
- colds
- sore throats

Rowan elixir
- colds
- rheumatism
- diarrhoea

[Diodgriafel, rowan ale, is] *made of the berries of* Sorbus Aucuparia, *(Roan Tree) abundant in most parts of Wales; by pouring water over them and setting the infusion by to ferment. When kept for some time, this is by no means an unpleasant liquor; but necessity obliges these children of penury to use it, without waiting for the fermentative process.*
– Evans (1798)

As a soft fruit it is … something of a failure, but, of course, it has one use which rescues it from foraging oblivion – Rowan jelly.
– Wright (2010)

[The berries] *are, however, terribly bitter but, as a Scottish friend once pointed out, they're our version of cranberry jelly, perfect for roasted meats.*
– Fowler (2011)

Rowan jelly

A traditional jelly, but nobody seems to agree on the balance of rowan berries and apples. We like equal amounts, and prefer crab apples to cooking apples. The apples or crab apples lighten the piquancy and their pectins help in the setting process.

Pick over and wash your **berries** and **apples**, quartering the latter; put both into a large pan, add **water** to cover and boil for some 20 minutes to a pulp. Allow to cool. Pour through a jelly bag and allow to drip overnight. Next day, measure the juice into a pan, and add 400g or 1lb **sugar** for each 500ml or 1 pint of **juice.** Heat slowly, stirring the sugar in until dissolved. Boil for 10 minutes or so, until a drop of the liquid solidifies when dribbled onto a cold saucer. Skim off the scum. Now pour into sterilised jars (heat in the oven for 10 minutes), cover and label.

Rowan syrup

Put 1kg (2.2lb) **rowan berries** into a pot, add **wate**r to cover and simmer until soft, about 25 minutes. Strain off the liquid, return berries to the pan and repeat with fresh water. This second boiling needs less time, roughly 15 minutes. Strain the liquid into a clean pan, add about ¾ caster (superfine) sugar to liquid (750g to 1 litre liquid). Boil hard for 5 minutes, then bottle in sterilised bottles. Label.

Rowan elixir

This heady elixir is made of equal parts of **vegetable glycerine** and **vodka** or **brandy**. Simply fill your jar with fresh-gathered and picked-over rowan berries, add the liquids, cover and leave in a dark place for at least six weeks. Strain off when the berries look bleached out.

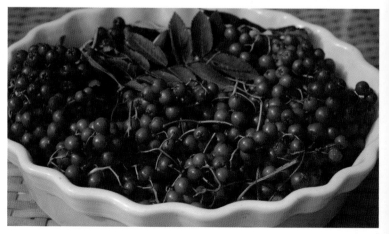

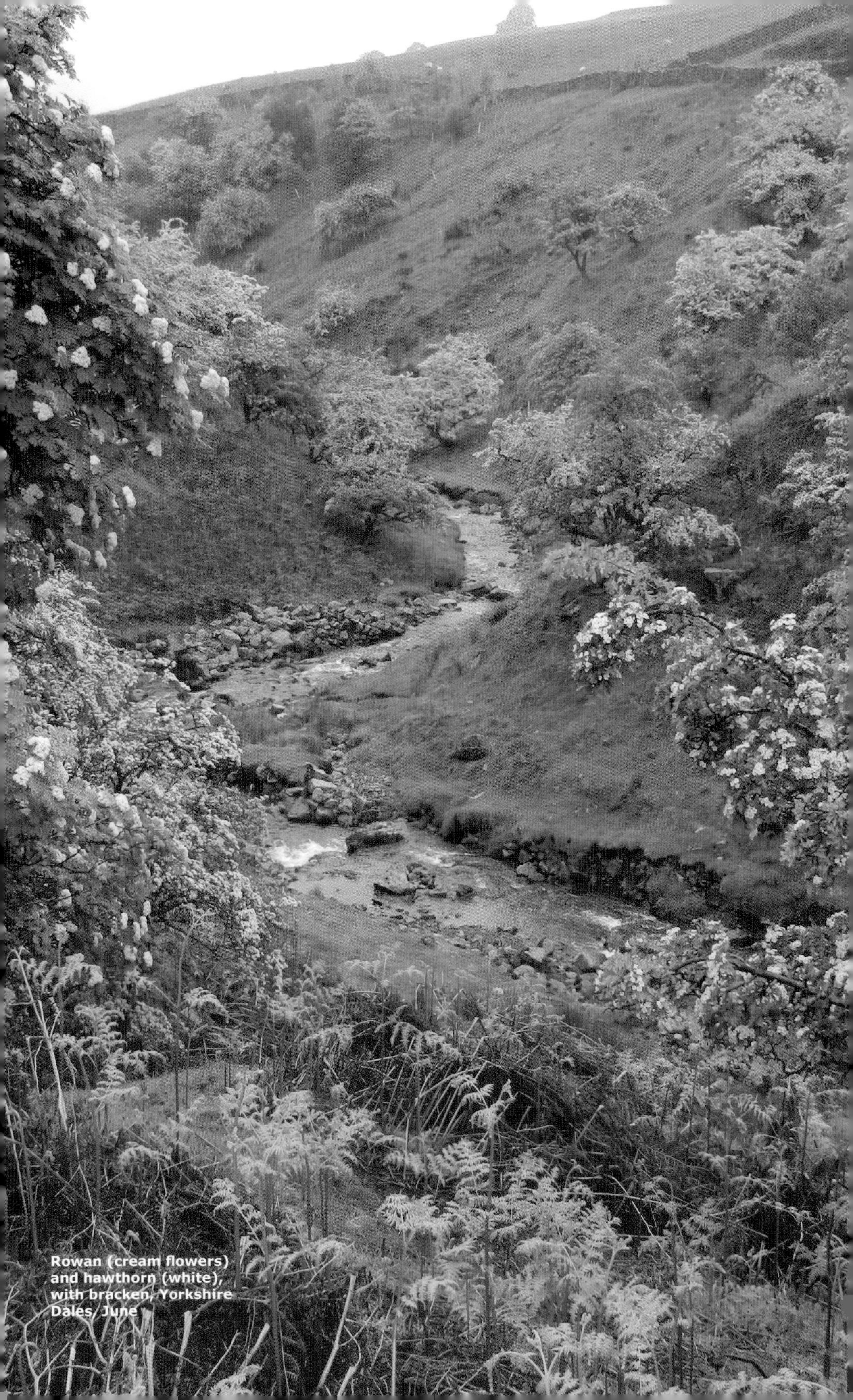

Rowan (cream flowers)
and hawthorn (white),
with bracken, Yorkshire
Dales, June

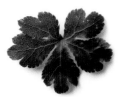

Sanicle Sanicula europaea

Sanicle is an easily overlooked woodland plant that was once regarded as a panacea, a cure-all, for healing wounds and uncontrolled bleeding, ulcers, tumours, and diseases of the mouth, throat, chest and lungs. It deserves to be better known for these uses and for its growing repute as an antiviral remedy.

Apiaceae
Carrot family

Description: A hairless perennial, some 60–70cm (2ft) high, with basal, palm-shaped, dark green 3- to 5-lobed leaves; the small puffs of white/pink flowers sit atop long stalks, often grouped 3 x 3, with a tenth central flower; fruit has hooked spines.

Habitat: Deciduous woodland, especially beechwoods on chalk, in colonies.

Distribution: Widespread in British Isles, Eurasia. *Sanicula marilandica* in North America.

Related species: Among the large Apiaceae family, sanicle is within a subfamily that includes masterwort or astrantia (*Astrantia major*) and sea holly (*Eryngo maritimum*). Common North American species are Canadian sanicle (*Sanicula canadensis*) and black sanicle or snakeroot (*S. marilandica*).

Parts used: Above-ground parts.

Sanicle (or wood sanicle in older herbals) is a forgotten and often overlooked plant of temperate deciduous woodland. It is one of those herbs that you never notice until it is pointed out to you, and then you see it everywhere.

When flowering in early summer sanicle's white/pink blossoms sit like ten or so pom-poms on top of a hairless stalk, more Allium than Apiaceae. Plantswoman Sarah Raven likens it to *a molecular model in a chemistry lab*.

A useful identifier is sanicle's preferred habitat – damp shade in old and usually coppiced woodland. Woodland authority Oliver Rackham (2006) includes it among 80 plant/tree indicators of ancient British woodland.

This habitat is under threat, as coppicing is in decline (which affects the shade regime) and as woodland is lost to development. The good news for sanicle fans is that, as we have found, it will grow readily in the garden, and make a good ground cover for shady areas.

Use sanicle for…
The common name has a connection with the Latin term 'to heal', and sanicle has a distinguished past as a medicinal, chiefly as a wound herb and anti-inflammatory for the chest and mouth. A medieval French saying summarises its reputation in ten words: *Celui qui Sanicle a / De plaie affaire il n'a* [who the Sanicle hath / At the surgeon may laugh].

Sanicle is one of the traditional European 'consounds' or wound herbs, and often linked with bugle (*Ajuga reptans*) and self-heal (*Prunella vulgaris*), both members of the deadnettle (Lamiaceae) family. Each of the three has been called 'self-heal' at some time. Comfrey is another 'consound'.

Geoffrey Grigson (1958) cites a 15th-century wound drink using leaves of sanicle, yarrow and bugle, crushed in a mortar and 'tempered with wine'. Each component had a subtle, complementary role: *This is the vertu of this drynke: bugle holdith the wound open, mylfoyle [yarrow] clensith the wound, sanycle helith it.*

Self-treatment for wounds was much more familiar in the past than now, but we believe it is valuable to know that herbs such as these (classed as vulneraries) can still be used as first aid. Sanicle works well for bruises and other minor injuries – simply chew a leaf to soften it, then apply to the injured area. If you are at home, you could also use a compress soaked in cooled sanicle tea and apply it to the skin.

Among other vulneraries or wound-healing herbs, including several common wild plants, are aloe vera, ashwagandha, burdock, calendula, comfrey, elder, garlic, plantain, St John's wort, thyme, woundwort and yarrow; tea tree essential oil can be added to this list, as can honey.

Sanicle is astringent and bitter, and had a long-standing reputation for dealing with irregular 'fluxes' or flows of bodily fluids. This extended from the blood, whether menstrual bleeding or ulcers, to disturbed urine or stool and upset stomachs. Sanicle tea is pleasant and can be drunk regularly to help heal internal ulcers.

Above all, sanicle was known as a treatment for the respiratory tract, as a gargle and mouthwash, for gum and throat problems, and for the lungs, including for tuberculosis. In North America, the local sanicle, *Sanicula marilandica*, was famed for treating sore throats and fevers.

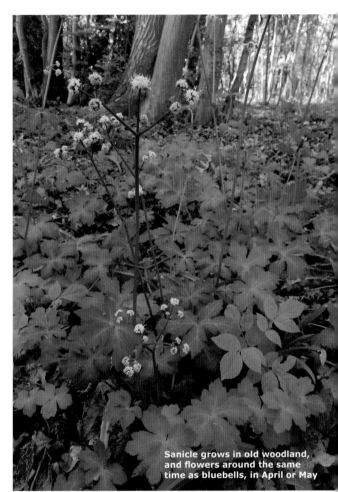

Sanicle grows in old woodland, and flowers around the same time as bluebells, in April or May

But sanicle's reputation has declined, particularly in the 20th century. We'd say this reflects broader medical changes (as in the standard treatment of tuberculosis) rather than any fault of the plant. The last great champion of sanicle was English herbalist Richard Lawrence Hool in the 1920s.

… there is not found any herbe [other than sanicle] that can give so much present helpe, either to man or beast, when the disease falleth upon the lunges or throate, and to heale up all the malignant putride or stinking ulcers of the mouth, throat, and privities.
– Parkinson (1640)

Hool's 1924 book features a sanicle tea to soothe ulcerated lungs or stomach. He suggests two parts sanicle to one part each of marshmallow and mullein in boiling water. The dosage is one or two glassfuls every three hours.

Hool also mentions a report in *Dr Skelton's Botanic Record* (1852) that a man had cured himself of consumption (tuberculosis) by drinking a pint daily of a tea of sanicle mixed with ginger, and then sweetened.

We propose that it is time that sanicle was not only identified in its woodland setting but also harvested, grown in the garden and used once again in medicine.

Modern research

A 1999 article confirmed antiviral effects for sanicle tea, with plaque inhibition shown in human parainfluenza virus type 2 (HPIV-2). An alcohol tincture of the plant did not have the same effect.

This complemented studies in 1996 by the same research team, which found that some kinds of influenza virus were disabled by sanicle extracts, without toxic effects on the subjects.

Research using the VOLKSMED database of traditional Austrian plant remedies (2013) found that sanicle was among 67 plants (of the 71 tested) to show anti-inflammatory activity *in vitro*, with 'moderate' to 'strong' effects.

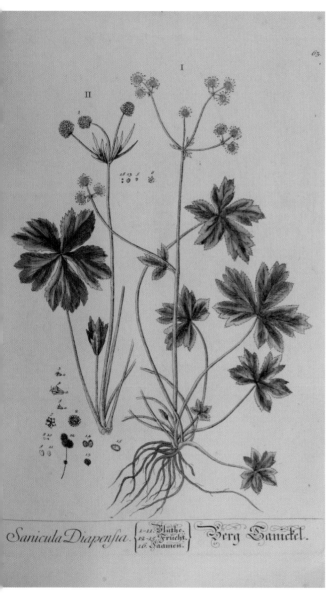

Sanicle, painted by Elizabeth Blackwell (1750), courtesy of the Wellcome Library

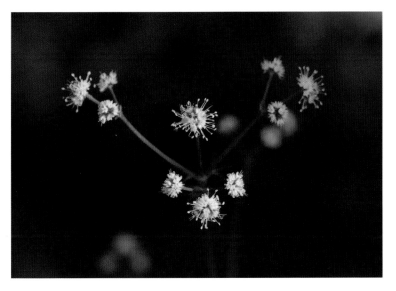

In cases of diseases of the chest and lungs, spitting of blood, scrofula, ulcers and tumours, or internal abscesses and ulcerations, there is no plant superior to Wood Sanicle.

– Hool (1924)

Wood sanicle has powerful medicinal properties and many uses. This is one of the herbs that could well be called a 'cure-all,' because it possesses powerful cleansing and healing virtue, both internally and externally. ... It is a powerful herb to heal both internal and external wounds and tumors [as a tea].

– Kloss (1939)

... vies for consideration as one of the most important but completely forgotten woundworts of the Middle Ages.

– Wood (2008)

Sanicle tea à la Parkinson

We tried John Parkinson's 1640 recipe for a sanicle tea. He states that the plant is astringent and bitter in taste, and suggests boiling fresh leaves and roots together, as a decoction, with 'a little hony put thereto'.

Two or three **sanicle leaves** per mug of **water** makes a good strong brew, with 10 or 15 minutes of gentle simmering until it turns golden. Then strain and add **honey** to taste. The honey not only makes the tea taste better, but adds to its effectiveness. The liquid can be bottled while hot or allowed to cool first, and keeps in the fridge for some weeks.

We found the initial effect to be relaxing, changing after a few minutes to stimulating. The energy is accompanied by a feeling of clarity, so you can decide what jobs need doing and then go ahead and finish them.

Sanicle flower essence

Julie made this essence with a shamanic friend, near the edge of an ancient woodland where there was a ploughed field just beyond. Sanicle strengthens our connection with the ancient magic of the forest, while providing strength and protection from external influences. It is both grounding and uplifting, and clarifies perception.

For full instructions on how to make a flower essence, see page 75 under forget-me-not.

Sanicle tea
- relaxing
- energising
- diarrhoea
- stomach upsets
- ulcers
- mouthwash
- sore gums
- lung problems

Sanicle essence
- connection
- strength
- protection
- intuition

Scabious

Field scabious, *Knautia arvensis*; Devil's bit scabious, *Succisa pratensis*

Scabious is perhaps best known as a garden border plant. Its pale lilac flowerheads are attractive to both humans and butterflies, it is easy to grow and has long stems that make it a good choice in flower arrangements. But did you know this was once a trusted wild-gathered plague herb?

Caprifoliacae Honeysuckle family

Description: Perennials, to 1m/3ft high (small scabious about half as tall); 'pincushion' purple-range flowerheads; devil's bit and sweet scabious are more rounded.

Habitat: Roadsides, woodland clearings, meadows; small scabious follows the chalk; devil's bit prefers damp, also heaths, fens.

Distribution: Europe and Middle East; devil's bit locally abundant in British Isles; field scabious common except for most of Scotland, central Wales, western Ireland; small scabious locally common, England only, mainly south and east; sweet scabious rare but for Kent and Cornwall. Field scabious is a widespread introduced species in the US.

Related species: Over 650 worldwide; many garden-bred.

Parts used: Whole plant, roots having strongest medicinal effect.

'Scabious' covers a number of pretty lilac or blue-flowered meadow plants, the most common of which are not within the Scabiosa genus. It's confusing!

In fact, the most frequently found scabiouses across the British Isles have other genus names: devil's bit scabious, or devil's bit, is *Succisa pratensis*, and field scabious, *Knautia arvensis*, is named for the German botanist Christopher Knaut (1638–94).

The true scabiouses – best known are the small scabious, *Scabiosa columbaria*, and the sweet scabious, *S. atropurpurea* – are at best locally common in the British Isles.

All four species are part of the wider scabious grouping for botanical and indeed medicinal purposes. Sheep's bit scabious, or sheep's bit (*Jasione montana*), however, is not a true scabious, despite its appearance. It is a *Campanula*, and not medicinal.

Modern reclassification has re-allocated the Scabious genus from the teasels to the honeysuckles. Field botanists might well hearken back to Linnaeus, who, in the mid-18th century, could name both *Knautia* and *Succisa* as *Scabiosa*!

As for 'scabious' itself, history offers two versions. First, the name comes from the Latin root-word *scabo*, meaning rough, as the hairy stem of field scabious might be described. More likely, perhaps, is the meaning for scab, mange or itch, describing some of scabious' medicinal properties. Perhaps the rough stalks were once used to rub the itch of scabies?

Geoffrey Grigson, for one, was unhappy with the English name. He wrote in 1958: *Scabious from the scab is a sad name for one of the most obvious, abundant, and pretty weeds of the cornfield. Perhaps one might abandon Scabious for 'Gipsy Rose'*.

No such luck yet, but there are other pleasing descriptive names from the past, for *Knautia* and *Succisa*: pincushion flower, blue bonnets, billy buttons, lady's hatpins and clodweed.

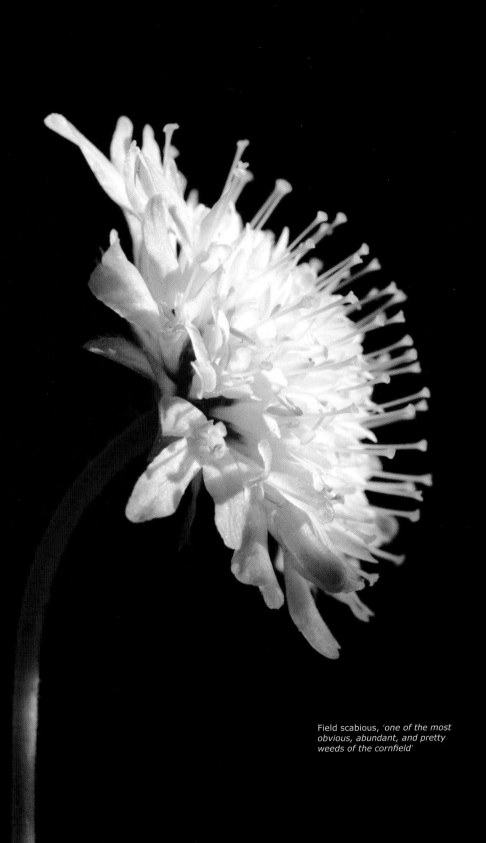

Field scabious, *'one of the most obvious, abundant, and pretty weeds of the cornfield'*

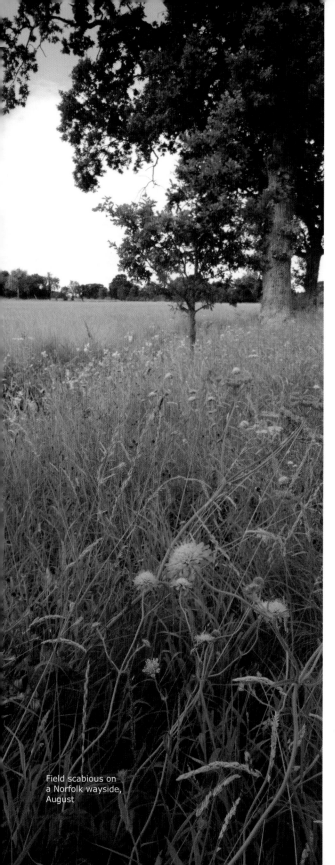

Field scabious on a Norfolk wayside, August

But there is one more name to mention, a remarkable one at that – devil's bit. This refers to the small truncated rootstock of the plant, which gave its former name *Morsus diaboli* or devil's bit(e). The story went that the root was so strong and good a medicine that the devil, 'envying the good that this herbe might do to mankinde', bit it off to destroy it.

Use scabious for…
Given this background, it will hardly be surprising that scabious root was a serious (if unavailing) treatment for plague and pestilence. The root was boiled in wine and the brew drunk, regularly, as a preventative. Its diaphoretic property helped patients sweat and break fevers.

The same remedy was used to treat bruising, dog bites and other blood wounds. The first book on distillation, the German alchemist Hieronymous Brunschwig's *Vertuous Book of Distillation* (1500), said an ounce of scabious water, drunk in the morning before food *is good for the pestilence*.

Additionally, the above-ground parts were crushed and laid on carbuncles, sores and itches, including scabies itself, to ripen and heal them. John Parkinson (writing in 1640) was confident that the bruised green herb of scabious, applied to a carbuncle or plague sore, *is found certaine by good experience* to dissolve or break it within three hours.

Parkinson's leading use for scabious, however, was as an expectorant for respiratory relief. He noted that devil's bit was the more bitter and stronger-acting of the scabious species. Both herbs could be made into syrups, decoctions or a distilled water.

By 1812, however, Hill's *Family Herbal* signposted the declining appeal of scabious. No longer a herb to fight the devil or the plague, for Hill it was a strong infusion for asthma, a syrup used for coughs and a juice applied on 'foulnesses of the skin'. Mrs Grieve in 1931 said much the same. But by 1979, Malcolm Stuart could write it off: *The herb* [Devil's bit scabious] *is not very effective medicinally and is rarely used today.*

But that marked a nadir, not an end. American herbalists like Matthew Wood and Peter Holmes are looking afresh at scabious. Wood, for example, in a workshop that Julie attended, reported herbalist Bernadette Dowling's finding that a long-brewed scabious tea was effective for relaxation. Holmes finds scabious has 'excellent topical applications', as in swabs, compresses and ointments; is good for bronchial issues and for various skin conditions. It's the sound of a wheel turning, not one halting.

Modern research
A scabious cousin, *Scabiosa arenaria*, in Tunisia (2015), was shown to inhibit α-glucosodase, a finding useful in type 2 diabetes treatment. Research on the same plant (2012) found its essential oil had antibacterial and anticandidal properties, comparable to those of thymol (the control).

In an ethnobotanical survey in rural Peru (2010), *Scabiosa atropurpurea* flowers were being used fresh orally or inhaled for menstrual regulation.

Scabious was in the past considered one of the finest remedies available for treating conditions affecting the skin. Like Plantain, Scabious addresses a large range of external conditions from wounds and abscesses to skin infections. ... Clearly this is another plant that deserves more widespread use in respiratory and topical applications.
– Holmes (2007)

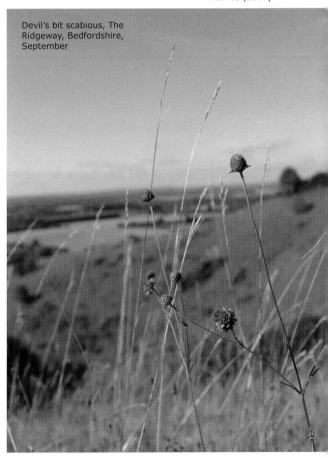

Devil's bit scabious, The Ridgeway, Bedfordshire, September

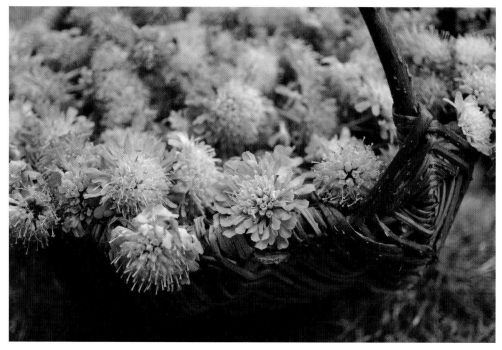

Scabious syrup

The inspiration for this recipe came from John Parkinson, who published his magnum opus, *Theatrum Botanicum*, in 1640.

Scabious syrup
- coughs
- asthma
- respiratory infections

Put a handful or two of **scabious** above-ground parts, fresh or dried, in a saucepan with 2 tablespoons chopped **liquorice root**, 2 tablespoons **fennel seed**, 1 tablespoon **aniseed** and 6 **dates**, chopped.

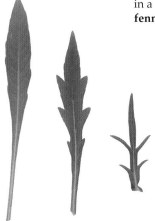

Add enough **water** to cover the herbs. Put the lid on the saucepan and bring to the boil, then remove from heat and cool overnight. The next day, strain the liquid into a clean saucepan, and gently simmer until reduced by about a third. Pour into a warmed sterile bottle. It has a rich, sweet flavour that masks any bitterness from the scabious.

Dose: Take 4 or 5 teaspoons a day, for respiratory issues.

Leaf progression of common scabious, from basal (left) to topmost leaves (right)

Sea buckthorn *Hippophae rhamnoides*

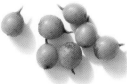

Sea buckthorn is a 'modern' herb, with an ancient Himalayan reputation but large-scale contemporary commercial exploitation. It is planted, especially in Central Asia and China, as a defence against desertification and erosion, and to fix sandy shores in Britain. Its vitamin- and antioxidant-rich orange berries are a superfood favourite; as well as skin and common cold treatments they have significant potential in elder health.

One recent September we picked and photographed the bright orange berries of sea buckthorn at Overstrand on the north Norfolk coast, and a few days later walked among the sea buckthorn specimens in the Mediterranean area at Kew Gardens.

Kew has many subspecies and cultivars of *Hippophae rhamnoides* (*Elaeagnus rhamnoides*) on show. Some were bushes and some trees up to 10m (33feet) high; they variously had thinner or thicker glaucous, willow-shaped leaves, and mostly bore smallish yellow or orange berries.

We agreed, after sampling and comparing as many berries as we could, that the most complex and satisfying taste came from the wild bush by the coast. Cultivation usually sweetens and simplifies flavour, and in this case the wild berries were larger and tangier.

Sea buckthorn berries are not easy to gather, because of the thorns and their squishiness if left too late, but are so well worth the effort. Choose your moment, and prepare for an experience that is intensely sweet, mixed with sourness, astringency and depth.

Winter migrant birds have always known the nutritious value of sea buckthorn berries, as did the ancient Greek, Chinese and Mongolian peoples. But no one knows whether the 'horse' element of the generic *Hippophae* name really refers to horses being given the berries to make their coat lustrous, as the original names suggest ('shining horse').

No matter, it is highly valued, and not only for the berries as food or medicine. Its roots grow fast and deep, stabilising sand and river banks, and are a first-line erosion and run-off defence in China. It is planted against desertification.

Moreover, the roots are also nitrogen-fixing, helping transform salty, sandy or acid soil into more fertile land for later crops. The density of the interlocked

Elaeagnaceae
Sea buckthorn family

Description: Spiny deciduous shrub, to 3m (10ft) tall, spreading vigorously by suckers, forming impenetrable thickets; narrow curling silvery leaves; flowers small, green, inconspicuous; they form plentiful green, later translucent orange berries, up to 1cm diameter, staying on the branch over winter.

Habitat: Sand dunes, sea shores as a rare British native; more commonly grown by roads, riverbanks, as an ornamental and to stabilise ground. Planted in deserts and mountains in Central and East Asia.

Distribution: Native in Europe, Russia, China. Introduced to Canada where it is called seaberry.

Related species: Spreading oleaster or autumn olive (*Elaeagnus umbellata*) is the only other British member of the family. Buckthorn (*Rhamnus cathartica*) and alder buckthorn (*Frangula alnus*) are in the unrelated Rhamnaceae, buckthorn, family.

Parts used: Berries, leaves.

branches and the profuseness of the thorns also quickly produce sea buckthorn thickets that form barriers to stock or human access and make efficient windbreaks.

This can be what is desired, but without rigorous maintenance can also become a runaway problem on the seashore and more so in civic planting – a pleasing show of berries in the autumn may well turn into an out-of-control jungle.

Use sea buckthorn for...
The first medicinal mention of sea buckthorn appears to be in a Tibetan text of the 8th century, where sea buckthorn ('rGyud bzi') features in 84 recipes.

Sea buckthorn's fame is much more recent, however, dating from the late 20th century, as is

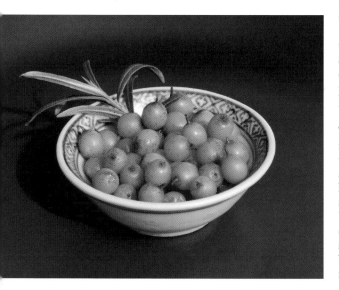

its separation from the buckthorn family and recognition as a separate genus. Buckthorn itself, *Rhamnus cathartica*, was formerly much more prized, as a purge. Parkinson's 1640 herbal, for example, scarcely mentions sea buckthorn or its berries.

But Parkinson does give an interesting recipe now long forgotten: *A decoction of the* [sea buckthorn] *leaves and inner barke thereof made in water whereunto a little allome* [alum] *is put is very good to wash the mouth when there is any inflammation or Ulcer or other disease therein.*

Modern emphasis is on sea buckthorn's rich resources of vitamins and minerals, in a heady cocktail of antioxidant benefits. The berries (and to a lesser extent the leaves) contain more vitamin C than oranges, more vitamin A (betacarotene) than carrots, high vitamin B2 and E; high omega 3 and 7; high potassium and quercetin; malic acid (giving the piquancy), flavonoids, unsaturated fatty acids, and so on.

The benefits are well advertised in many commercial products. We will pass by the claimed cancer and cardiovascular benefits, and highlight anti-inflammatory action and skin protection from UV radiation and free radical damage, via a sea buckthorn oil or sunscreen. The oil is said to have been used after the Chernobyl reactor disaster (1986) to treat radiation burns. It is more usually applied in the unsettling skin conditions psoriasis and eczema.

In this, there is a continuity here with older practice: Parkinson's list of skin conditions so treated in his time included *Saint Anthonies fire* [erysipelas] *and other fretting and eating Cankers* [cancers]… *pushes, wheales* [skin eruptions] *etc.*

Sea buckthorn oil – commercially made from the seeds, pulp or whole fruit – is easily absorbed by the skin, and the omega 7s strongly support mucous membranes and skin lipids. The berries' high vitamin C helps combat the common cold, in building resistance and as a prophylactic. Mixed with rose hips it is more palatable for children.

The benefit we will focus on, however, is sea buckthorn's dramatic end-of-options curative power and for convalescence. For example, an occasional whole berry helped Julie through six weeks of recovery and kept further infection at bay.

Regular use of the berries is said to protect against arteriosclerosis and improve the eyesight by assisting microcirculation. The berries are said to ease the menopause and to help maintain cognitive health. In other words, sea buckthorn should be promoted to the list of outstanding herbs, and wild ones at that, for elder health. Moreover it is a safe and long-term remedy.

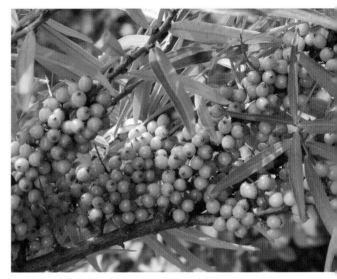

Modern research

Sea buckthorn capsules have become a well-known health supplement and superfood, sold online and in health shops.

The juice meanwhile has become a superfood trend. It was identified as an element of 'cutting-edge New Nordic cuisine' in a 2016 US press report. Expect to find it in 'healthy' cocktails and smoothies for a year or two yet. Perhaps the next taste will be a literal version of its old folk name 'Siberian pineapple'?

It has also been the subject of a surge of research in the present century, well summarised in a 2012 'remedial prospective'.

Among the more specific medicinal studies are a human trial in 2006 in which the oil eaten

The berries are very abundant, on short peduncles, ovate, or ovate-globular … red or yellow when ripe, succulent, smooth … gratefully acid, and are much eaten by the Tartars.
– Wilkes (1811)

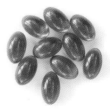

Sea buckthorn oil capsules

in porridge reduced risk factors of cardiovascular disease. A 2011 study on rats showed that the oil lessened cardiotoxicity.

The seed oil showed 'significant' wound-healing activity on rats with induced burns (2009), and it was a 'hopeful drug' for the prevention and treatment of liver fibrosis in other research (2003). A sea buckthorn wine intended to treat oxidative stress and hypercholesterolemia has been made (2013), and a herb tea from the leaves and twigs shows high rutin and antioxidative content (2016).

Harvesting sea buckthorn

What you need is the whole berries or their juice. Wear protective gauntlets against the thorns, and take care. It is easiest to collect by lifting the berries with a fork into a container, such as a plastic sandwich box. It will be messy, with unwanted bits of leaf and twigs, but these can be strained off at home. And think of the bracing sea air!

Some foragers advocate cutting off whole fruit-bearing branches and taking them home, until needed, but you should have express permission of the landowner to butcher the plant like this. It may be feasible where the thickets have overgrown and need clearing.

Store the berries or 'mush' in the fridge until needed; freezing will sweeten the overall taste (a process known as 'bletting').

Sea buckthorn kefir

Add 2 tablespoons **water kefir grains** and ¼ cup **light brown sugar** per litre of **water**. Leave to ferment for about 48 hours, then strain out the

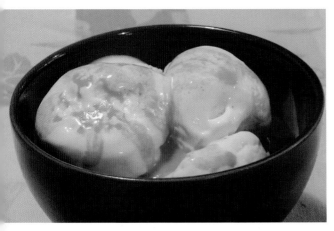

grains and pour the liquid into bottles. Fill each litre bottle ¾ full, then top up with **apple juice** and 1 to 2 tablespoons of **sea buckthorn juice**. It's ready to drink as soon as it becomes slightly fizzy, usually after 24 to 48 hours depending on the temperature and other factors.

Sea buckthorn with ice cream

One of the easiest and most delicious ways to use sea buckthorn is to pour the juice over your vanilla ice cream or glacé.

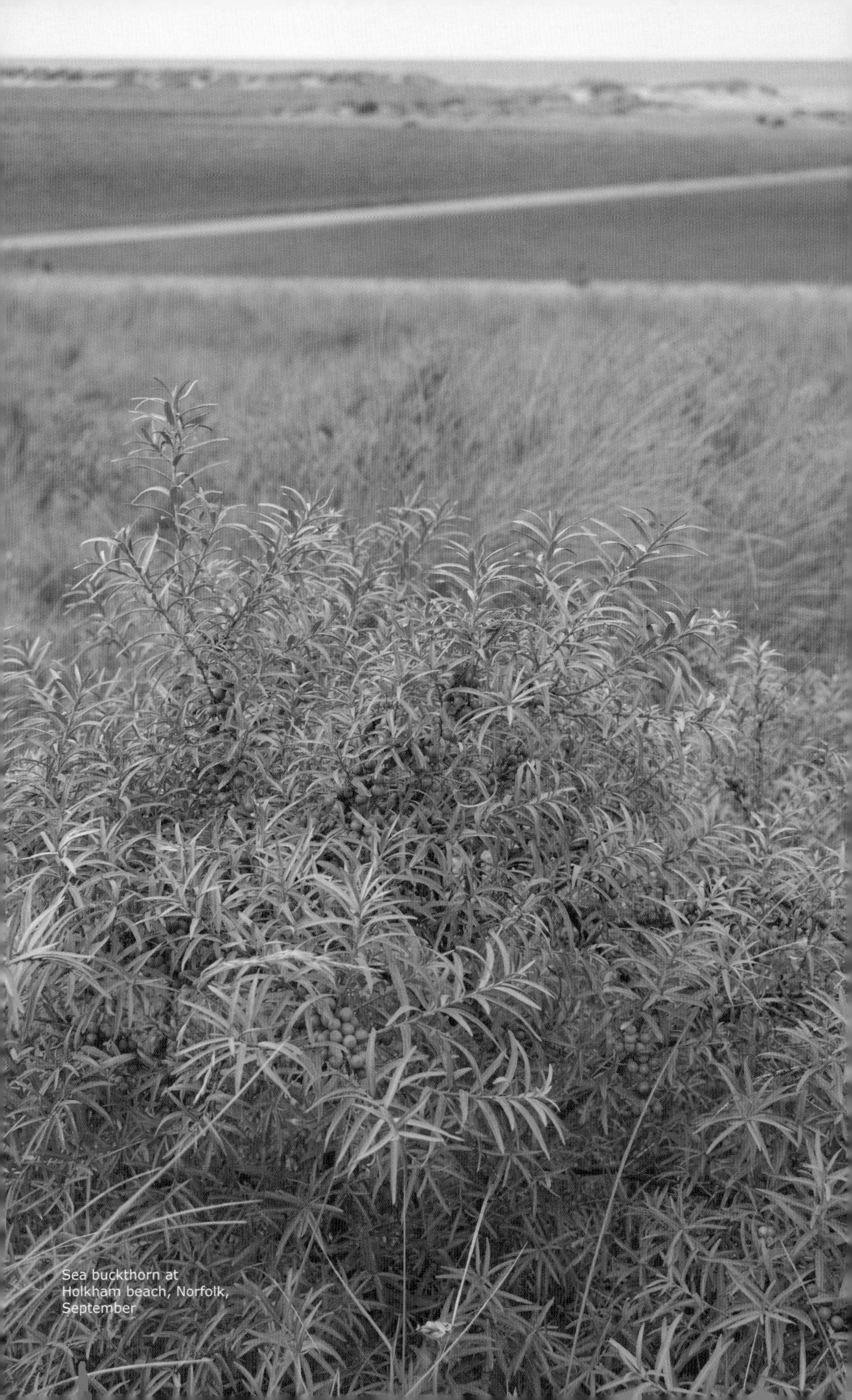

Sea buckthorn at
Holkham beach, Norfolk,
September

Silverweed *Potentilla anserina*
Tormentil *Potentilla erecta*
Cinquefoil *Potentilla reptans*

**Rosaceae
Rose family**

Description: Tormentil is generally erect, the other two are creeping; all have bright yellow flowers, with 5 petals, except for tormentil, usually with 4; silverweed leaves are distinctive; all have knobbly rootstocks, thickest, hardest and reddest in tormentil.

Habitat: All three similar: waysides, dunes, open woodland, while tormentil also favours heath and bog.

Distribution: All three widely distributed through the British Isles. Mainly in northern hemisphere; native to Europe and western Asia; silverweed native to North America, introduced to Australasia.

Related species: Near-relatives of agrimony and avens (also Rose family), with similar medicinal profiles as astringents.

Parts used: Leaves and flowers for silverweed and cinquefoil, roots for tormentil.

These three Potentilla species are the best-known medicinal plants in the genus, and have largely overlapping uses. Known since ancient Greek times for treating colitis, diarrhoea and mouth issues, they are strong astringents whose traditional but generally overlooked benefits are attracting new interest.

The Potentillas are a genus in the rose family, with some 17 species and subspecies in Britain, about 75 in Europe, and over 300 worldwide. The numbers are approximate because of the ease with which the Potentillas hybridise – a botanist's challenge, if not a nightmare – and with ongoing reclassification issues.

But those who practise wayside medicine are lucky in that the three leading medicinal Potentillas are readily recognisable. The genus name translates as 'little powerful one', and the reference is to medicinal potency, which we can now ascribe to high tannin content and resulting astringency.

Tormentil varies in height, being shorter in open heathland and taller in shaded woodland, but it is the one species that typically has four yellow petals. The other Potentillas usually have five, but silverweed is the only species to have silver-green foliage, especially noticeable below its

saw-tooth leaves. Cinquefoil or five-leaf grass has the usual five petals and leaves but also stretchy stolons, which can be a metre long.

Tormentil, *Potentilla erecta*, has also been known as blood root and tormenting root. The unusual English name is from medieval Latin *tormina*, meaning both colitis and the pain or torment it causes; some say it referred to the pain of toothache. Tormentil root, then, was taken to ease these unpleasant conditions – and still can be.

Julie's tormentil tincture is blood red, goes straight to the back of

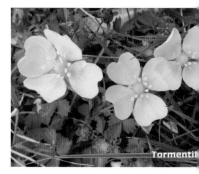

Tormentil

the throat and is very dry and astringent (Sir John Hill in 1812 called the effect 'austere'). It feels exactly right for treating throat and mouth issues.

The tannins are unusually high (sometimes over 20% of the physical constituents), enough to make tormentil roots useful in tanning leather, particularly in areas where oak trees are scarce.

Silverweed, *Potentilla anserina*, has other attractive names, such as prince's feathers, Argentina, fish bones, goosewort, goose tansy, bread and cheese, traveller's ease.

Most are explained by the leaf colour or plume-like form. *Argentina* is from *argent*, Latin for silver. *Anserina* means 'goose-like', for the way geese love to eat it (as do most stock animals, except for sheep). Traveller's ease is for an old use of leaves as a shoe lining.

Silverweed roots have been a significant famine food, from the Western Isles of Scotland to the Pacific Northwest of America. We love the tender, floury flavour of the boiled roots. The plant was so frequent in sandy shores that it was sometimes actively farmed, and dug up with ploughs.

As a source of starch, roots can be boiled or roasted and ground into flour, for bread or porridge. The 19th-century folklorist Alexander Carmichael called silverweed 'one of the seven breads of the Gael'.

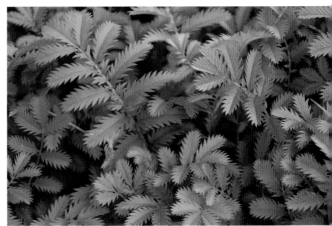

John Ray in 1670 thought they tasted like parsnips; John Wright in 2010 suggests chestnuts or Jerusalem artichokes.

Cinquefoil, *Potentilla reptans* (literally creeping cinquefoil), was also known as five-leaf grass – Mrs Grieve, as late as 1931, used this common name as her main heading. Other country names she reports include five-finger blossom, golden blossom and St Anthony's turnip.

Cinquefoil is aggressive, its reddish runners (stolons) making vigorous ground cover in bare ground, waysides and woodlands. It is an ancient companion of man. It seems that cinquefoil is the original Potentilla described by the Greek herbalist Dioscorides in the 1st century AD as *Pentaphyllon* (five leaves), and whose qualities as a fever remedy he espoused. Already in his time it was an anti-malarial herb in Egypt.

Silverweed leaves, above, and flower, below

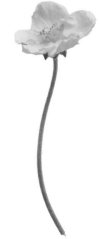

[Tormentil and silverweed] ... *are two varieties of* Potentilla *and can be used interchangeably. However, Silverweed root ... is also an intestinal relaxant/ spasmolytic, and is also called Crampwort.*
– Holmes (2006)

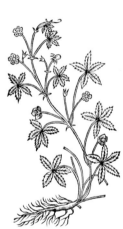

Cinquefoil, woodcut from Parkinson, *Theatrum Botanicum* (1640)

Use silverweed, tormentil and cinquefoil for...

The medicinal uses of these closely related species are largely interchangeable. French herbalist Jean Palaiseul calls them the 'potentil sisters'. Internally, the trio work effectively on 'tormenting' conditions such as acute diarrhoea and dysentery, colitis (both mucous and ulcerative forms), peptic and gastric ulcers, irritable bowel and Crohn's disease.

The astringent effect (most profound in **tormentil**) involves coating vessel membranes with a protective layer, being antiseptic to inflammation and helping stop discharges. John Pechey noted in 1707: *It dries, and is very astringent; wherefore there is no Remedy more proper for Fluxes of the Belly and Womb, than the Roots of Tormentil.*

Externally, a decoction or lotion of all three plants helps stop local bleeding in cuts and piles, or vaginal discharge; is soothing for sores, burns, sunburn or frostbite; and makes an excellent gargle for any throat or mouth-based inflammations. In addition to the tea as a drink, compresses soaked in it can be applied to sore places.

This broad range of treatment possibilities makes the Potentillas a very useful family to know for long-distance walkers and campers: whether facing sunburn or windburn, rucksack rash or saddle-sore pack animals, grazes, sore feet or gippy tummy, you are likely to have help at close hand. Chewing at the very hard root of tormentil or the other plants is good emergency relief for sore gums, toothache or mouth ulcers.

Specifically, **silverweed** is most used as a mouthwash, for sore gums and loose teeth, and is gentle enough (having more mucilage) for a baby's teething. Mixed with milk, it was popularly thought to remove freckles and lighten a sunburned complexion. A country name for silverweed, in Britain and the USA, is cramp weed, and the tea is excellent for a cramping stomach.

Supplementing its generic qualities, **cinquefoil** has a specialism as an intermittent fever remedy, as in ague or malaria.

All three plants are considered safe and non-toxic, but long-term use should be approached cautiously, especially for people suffering from persistent diarrhoeal-type issues.

Modern research

A 2009 study of *P. erecta* rhizomes on rats and mice showed no toxicity in strong dosages, confirming recent clinical human trials. These found no toxicity in using tormentil to treat ulcerative colitis in adults and rotavirus-induced diarrhoea in children.

In a major review (2014a), herbal treatments of ulcerative colitis (aloe vera gel, *P. erecta* extracts, wheat grass juice and curcumin) were assessed. Tormentil extracts at 2,400mg per day halved the clinical activity index and C-reactive protein levels of 16 patients, without side effects.

In 2003, 40 children, aged from 3 months to 7 years with rotavirus diarrhoea were given *P. erecta* drops, which cut duration of the diarrhoea to 3 days (placebo 5).

A study (2014b) found that four Potentilla species all showed free radical-scavenging effect (DPPH), and influenced the viability and cytokine production of colon cell walls. Nine Potentilla species had proven antibacterial effects, notably against *H. pylori* (2008).

A 2011 study was the first to look at the *in vitro* inhibitory effects of *P. erecta* aerial parts extracts against cariogenic *Streptococcus* spp. strains in the human oral environment. Results suggested plant efficacy as a possible supplement for pharmaceutical products presently used for mouth care.

It [tormentil] *is considered one of the safest and most powerful of our native aromatic astringents, and for its tonic properties has been termed 'English Sarsaparilla'.*
– Grieve (1931)

Of all the many astringents available I find small doses of this one [tormentil] *almost irreplaceable in the treatment of peptic, especially gastric ulcers.*
– Barker (2001)

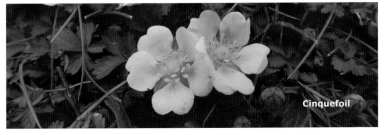
Cinquefoil

Potentilla root wine

We used cinquefoil root because it is our local abundant species, but tormentil or silverweed can be used the same way. Cinquefoil has a taproot with a swollen node at the top.

Pour 1 cup **white wine** into a small saucepan. Add a small handful of chopped cinquefoil **roots**, a couple of **cloves**, and a small piece of **cinnamon** stick. Simmer gently with the lid on for about 15 minutes, then remove from heat, add a teaspoon or two of **honey** and leave to cool. Bottle and label.

Take a small wineglassful three times a day for convalescence and weakness after an illness. It can also be used as a mouth rinse for gum problems.

Potentilla root wine
- convalescence
- gum problems
- mouth ulcers
- loose bowels
- heavy periods

Silverweed root sauté

Break off the swollen roots of **silverweed**, and simmer in a little **water** until tender. Sauté with butter or oil.

Sowthistle *Sonchus* spp.

Asteraceae
Daisy family

Description: Smooth sowthistle (*Sonchus oleraceus*) has smooth grey-green matt leaves and pale yellow flowers; prickly sowthistle (*S. asper*) is similar but with darker green and spiny 'thistly' leaves; perennial sowthistle (*S. arvensis*) is straggly with golden hairs and deep yellow flowers in late summer and autumn. Height depends on habitat.

Habitat: All three species like disturbed ground, arable fields, waysides; smooth sowthistle often found in gardens (and flowers in mild winters), perennial sowthistle on shorelines and riversides.

Distribution: All three species abundant across whole of British Isles except for the Scottish Highlands. Found worldwide, and classed as invasive in the US and Canada.

Related species: Marsh sowthistle (*S. palustris*) is a locally common fenland species in eastern England; can grow to 3m (10ft) tall.

Parts used: Stems and their latex, leaves, flowering tops; roots used in Asia.

The sowthistles comprise some 60 species worldwide, three of which are native to Europe and the Middle East, and have readily spread to temperate regions around the world. They are known, variously vilified or valued, as invasive arable weeds, foraged food and as a largely forgotten medicinal.

In terms of kinship, appearance and usefulness the sowthistles (genus *Sonchus*) lie somewhere between the dandelions and thistles. All are members of the vast Asteraceae or daisy family.

Julie remembers being made aware of the culinary possibilities of sowthistle by a passage from Margaret Roberts (1983) on its use in South Africa: *The Tswanas on our farm gather* [sowthistle] *from the mealieland* [corn] *edges and feed it to their pigs. In times of vegetable scarcity they make a mild and pleasant spinach-like dish from the young leaves and flowering tops, flavoured with chopped onion.*

But the reputation of sowthistles is mixed. Edible plant collector and grower Stephen Barstow points out they are classified as weeds in over a quarter of all countries (some 55 of 193 in the United Nations). Yet sowthistle is *just about the most useful vegetable in my garden* for most of his growing season.

Arthur Lee Jacobson, an American herb blogger, adds: *Sow Thistles are close cousins of lettuces, and the best*

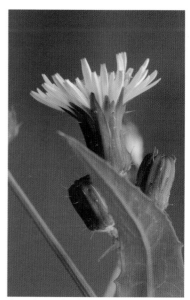

Smooth sowthistle

specimens are described more truly as wild salad herbs than as loathsome weeds. Taste the greens and maybe you'll agree.

The perennial sowthistle (*S. arvensis*) is an opportunist, pioneer plant and is thought to be an early coloniser after the retreat of the ice caps; it readily grows after fires, volcanoes, earthquakes and bombs; and in almost any soil, even in cracks in concrete. Modern farmers know it reproduces from root fragments after ploughing as well as from its seed parachutes.

The sowthistles are an ancient food and medicine, with British archaeological records from the Bronze Age in Derbyshire. It was certainly familiar in ancient Greece and Rome. Pliny tells a legend of Theseus, who was given a meal of sowthistle leaves by a poor peasant lady, Hecale, on his way to capture the Bull of Marathon.

It has not escaped modern commentators that this is akin to Popeye and his spinach, the leaves endowing the underdog hero with powers of courage and strength. As a green forage food sowthistle is found in most contemporary cultures of temperate regions, from *kucai* in China to *preboggión* in Italy, from *puwha* of the Maori of New Zealand to *morogo* or *imifino* in South Africa. This should hardly be surprising given that *oleraceus* (as in smooth sowthistle) means 'edible'.

It was noted by Pliny (1st century AD) as an everyday salad and vegetable item, and is still an ingredient in *insalata di campo* (field salad) in northern Italy, alongside chicory and dandelion. The related alpine blue sowthistle (*Cicerbita alpina*) is such a delicacy in the Trento and Veneto regions that its picking has had to be regulated.

Sowthistle is part of the Passover seder meal in Israel. Described as *maror* (bitter), it symbolises the bitterness of Jewish slavery.

In a less solemn context, American forager 'Wildman' Steve Brill says he can always count on sow thistles for the 'Wildman's Five-Boro Salad' featured at his mid-December annual Wild Party in New York. He comments that it is an appropriate dish for this event, since some guests eat like pigs!

So, is sowthistle animal or human food? It is both. It is sought out by pigs and fed to pigs, but has also been called dog's thistle, hare's lettuce and rabbit's meat. Various animals – chickens and cage birds too – know it is good for them.

The botanist John Ray had a view on this. He noted in 1690 that some people used sowthistle as a winter vegetable with salad, but *We leave it to be masticated by hares and rabbits.* That may be Ray's loss, because the cooked leaves taste sweetish, nutty and flavoursome.

Use sowthistle for...
The genus name *Sonchus* means hollow, referring to the stems. The stems of all species have a milky latex or juice, which has inspired popular names of milkwort, milkweed and milk thistle (all of these are distinct from milk thistle per se, *Silybum marianum*).

The juice is traditionally a wart medicine, as are most latex

[Common sowthistle] *is quoted as one of the world's worst weed plants and is said to be a pest in at least 55 countries. But to me, this is just about the most useful vegetable in my garden from late spring when the perennials are finished to late autumn. Do as I do, FEST ON PESTS!* – Barstow (2014)

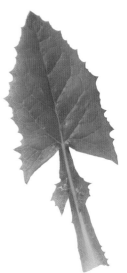

Smooth sowthistle leaf

*Sow thistle may be a common weed throughout South Africa, but it is one with such healing properties that one is very pleased to see its appearance every year.
– Roberts (1983)*

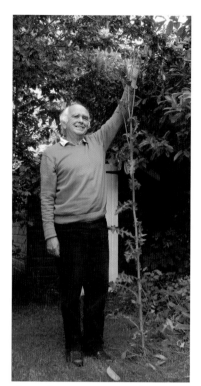

Matthew standing by a very tall prickly sowthistle in our garden, June

Coming closer to the present day, sowthistle was used by Chinese residents in early 1900s San Francisco, where it was said to benefit opium users trying to break their addiction. This finding requires modern examination, but sowthistle does have a reputation for treating addiction and anxiety in general.

Recent research explains sowthistle as protective for the liver and kidneys through its polyphenol content, with free radical-scavenging properties. This is reflected in a former reputation as a hepatitis herb. In Nepal the juice of the root is used to clear the bile ducts.

One traditional use that has modern support is for using the latex diluted in a liquid to treat cough, asthma and bronchitis. Parkinson again: *the milke that is taken from the stalkes when they are broken, given in drinke, is beneficial to those that are shortwinded and have a weesing withall.*

A final recommendation from Parkinson is that the distilled water of sowthistle is fit for 'the daintiest stomach' and is 'wonderfully good' as a face wash.

In China the local sowthistle is used by older people for maintaining vitality and virility; it has been used clinically for erectile dysfunction, and for 'strangury' (small quantities of urine) or dysuria (painful urination).

plants. It was seen as cooling in herbal action, and John Parkinson (1640) notes that *the herbe bruised or the juyce is profitably applied to all hot inflammations in the eyes, or wheresoever else.* It yielded a soothing salve applied on hot skin eruptions of various kinds, and can still be used in this way. The leaves were poulticed for the same purpose, and applied to wounds or to bring down fevers.

Parkinson adds another virtue now forgotten: *the juyce boyled is a sure remedy for deafnesse and singings and all other diseases in the ears.*

Modern research

If older uses of sowthistle are impressive and perhaps should never have been forgotten, white-coat research is adding some remarkable potential extensions.

In significant New Zealand findings Thompson & Shaw (2002) show that use of sowthistle (and/or watercress) in Maori diets may reduce their colorectal cancer levels, compared with non-Maori peoples. The figures per 100,000 people were 22.2 for Maoris and 43.7 for non-Maoris. Disadvantaged in most lifestyle indices, the Maori were nonetheless at lower risk of this form of cancer, and use of these plants in their diet appeared to be the decisive factor.

Research in Pakistan (2012) confirmed that *S. asper* was protective against potassium chromate ingestion that led to male sexual dysfunction in rats. Other findings by the same team (2011) demonstrated that the same plant had 'remarkable capacity to scavenge' and its antioxidant phytochemicals lent it potential as a medicine against free radical-associated oxidative damage, especially in the liver and kidneys.

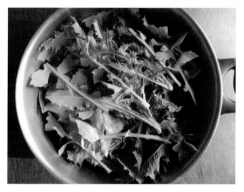

Harvesting sowthistle

Sowthistle can be harvested much of the year. We love eating the succulent flower buds, best picked when the first few flowers are opening. For eating the leaves, smooth sowthistle is best, but the leaves of prickly sowthistle can be used if the spines along the edges are trimmed off – easy with a pair of scissors. The pot above (left) contains both species.

Sowthistle pakora

Collect a few handfuls of sowthistle leaves or flower buds. Mix 250g/½ lb **gram** (chickpea flour), 1 teaspoon **baking powder** and ½ teaspoon **salt**, then stir in enough **water** to make a batter. Add your chopped-up **sowthistle**, and mix into the batter. Heat **vegetable oil** for deep frying. Drop tablespoons of the mixture into the hot oil and fry until golden, then drain. Eat while hot.

Speedwell
Veronica officinalis, V. beccabunga, V. chamaedrys, V. serpyllifolia

The speedwells look like tiny waifs and strays of the wayside flora, their bright blue flowers optimistic and pleasing. Actually they are tough wild survivors, once valued in mainstream European herbalism as a panacea and returning to favour for treating inflammations, nervous exhaustion and whooping cough.

**Plantaginaceae
Plantain family**

Description: Generally low-lying (to 50cm, 20in), mostly perennial herbs, usually with opposite leaves, round stems and attractive blue or violet spectrum four-petalled flowers either at tip or in leaf axils of the stem.

Habitat: Usually dry meadows, hedgerows and gardens, though brooklime grows in streams and some scarcer species are found in the Breckland heaths of East Anglia.

Distribution: Native to Europe, Western Asia, and naturalised in North America and Australasia.

Related species: The common wild British speedwells include brooklime (*Veronica beccabunga*) and the following speedwells: common field (*V. persica*), germander (*V. chamaedrys*), heath (*V. officinalis*), ivy-leaved (*V. hederofolia*), marsh (*V. scutellata*), slender (*V. filiformis*), thyme-leaved (*V. serpyllifolia*) and wall (*V. arvensis*).

Parts used: Above-ground parts.

The Veronicas or speedwells were once included in the figwort family (Scrophulariaceae) but are now classed as plantains (Plantaginaceae). Whatever their designation they remain small, eye-catching and sparky. As Mrs Grieve notes, the Veronica genus *contains some of our most beautiful native flowers, the speedwells*.

There are some 500 speedwell species worldwide, with about 27 in the British Isles, nine of which can be regarded as common (see related species). We focus on four: the 'official' or heath speedwell, brooklime, germander and thyme-leaved speedwell. We will treat them together, and propose that thyme-leaved speedwell should be added to the other more common species as a useful medicinal.

Our interest was piqued in a recent year when it seemed that speedwells were pursuing us. We were searching for heath speedwell, the official species used in medicine, but instead everywhere we went we found the similar but tiny thyme-leaved speedwell growing. We even

returned home and found it abounding in our own garden, in plant pots and in the lawn, which hadn't been mown while we were away!

Why the nudges? To get in the mood to answer that we try out a spoonful each of a tincture of thyme-leaved speedwell made that summer.

First impression is of a light, aromatic, aniseedy taste, with a touch of sweet astringency. It goes straight to the third eye, leaving a euphoric, eye-cleaning sensation and a slight buzziness. After about two minutes the focus descends and spreads out, feeling like a spirit of goodwill that warms and wakens you up – not just in the heart, but the body as a whole.

It's rather wonderful, a calming yet uplifting sensation – maybe speedwells are to be understood as spiritual herbs operating on the UV spectrum, or have their physical uses just been replaced and forgotten? In any case we thought the plants were telling us something.

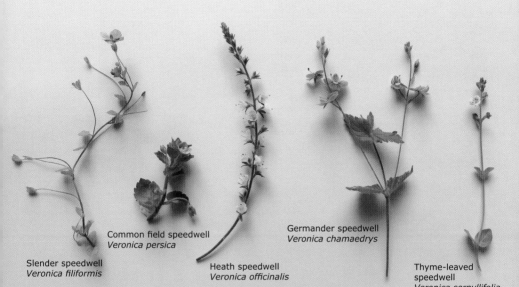

Common field speedwell
Veronica persica

Germander speedwell
Veronica chamaedrys

Slender speedwell
Veronica filiformis

Heath speedwell
Veronica officinalis

Thyme-leaved
speedwell
Veronica serpyllifolia

We did finally find heath speedwell growing, in Ireland, first in the Burren, then at Loughcrew on 2 July – the year's 182/183-day tipping point – there it was, official speedwell growing abundantly in the grass.

The common name 'speedwell' bears an old meaning of 'thrive' or 'get better', as in 'speed you well' or 'God speed'. The more formal 'Veronica' might derive from the Latin words *vero* and *eikon*, meaning 'true image'.

One story relates that a woman, later St Veronica, bathed the face of Christ as he carried the Cross, and the image left on the cloth resembled patterns on the flowers. This visage may not be clearly apparent, but do look at speedwell flowers with a hand lens. Observe their intricacy – the white border outside the deep azure blue of germander and its 'bird's eye' central white spot; the tiny leaves of thyme-leaved speedwell; the bright blue flowers and succulent, dark stems of brooklime; the pale violet petals with darker lines of heath speedwell, and so on.

Another rendering of 'Veronica' is from the Greek *phero* and *nike*, meaning 'I bring victory', referring to its plant's medicinal usefulness.

Take these name explanations for what they are worth, but there is no doubt that speedwells were cultivated in monastic gardens, and for centuries were

Identifying the most widespread British terrestrial speedwells

This little herb [Heath speedwell] *has wonderful healing properties seemingly out of all proportion to its size.*
– Roberts (1983)

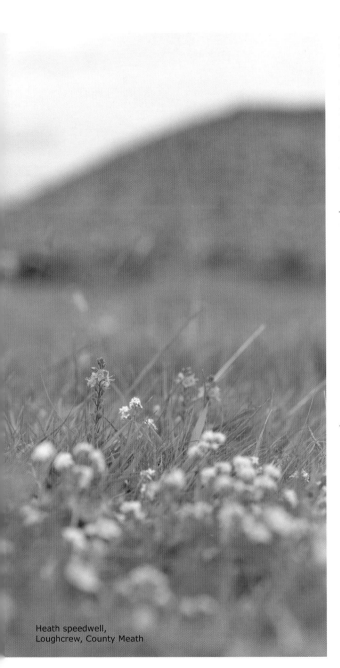

Heath speedwell,
Loughcrew, County Meath

part of mainstream European herbalism. The speedwells were valued, almost as a panacea, as expectorants for treating bronchitis and asthma, arthritis and rheumatism, for haemorrhages, for skin, liver and kidneys, and externally as wound herbs.

John Parkinson (1640) ascribed strong 'virtues' to the speedwell family, as *a singular good remedy for the Plague, and all Pestilentiall Fevers*, for leprosy, for *all manner of coughes and diseases of the brest and lunges*, for opening obstructions of the liver and spleen, for kidney stone and various tumours.

In 1690, heath speedwell was the subject of a 300-page monograph by Johannes Francke, the *Polychresta Herba Veronica*. Shortly thereafter John Pechey (in 1694, and a second edition in 1707) related how a *large Dose of the* [speedwell] *Decoction, taken for some time* expelled a kidney stone that a woman had had for sixteen years; a speedwell poultice removed the inflammation of 'an incurable Ulcer' in a man's leg; and the distilled water cured a woman's 'Fistula in the Breast'.

By the 19th century, however, speedwell had declined in medicinal regard and was mostly used as a tea substitute, known in France as *thé d'Europe*. The great Linnaeus in the previous century said he preferred this to black tea. We find it very restorative when we are feeling weary and tired.

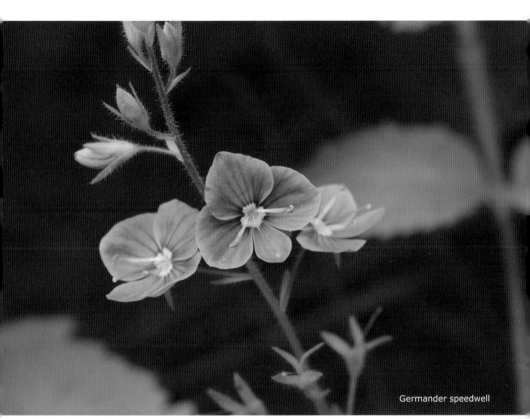
Germander speedwell

British herbalist Julian Barker summarises: *From its heady days of the 16th and 17th centuries where it was vaunted as panacea for all manner of digestive and respiratory troubles, including TB, it has slipped into the position, if remembered at all, of a good domestic beverage and digestive aid.*

This status was exacerbated in 1935 when the French botanist and systematiser of phytotherapy, Henri Leclerc, stated his opinion that speedwell tea was no more useful than the hot water used to make it. But this was a low point. Maria Treben in Austria and Margaret Roberts in South Africa, among others, have since championed speedwell and advocated its reintroduction into contemporary herbal medicine. We couldn't agree more.

Use speedwells for...
Treben points out that the Romans learned of speedwell from the Teutons, and it was a Roman compliment to say that someone has *as many good qualities as a speedwell.*

Only time and further research will tell whether it was right to drop this herb [Heath speedwell] *from our materia medica.*
– Hatfield (2007)

We suggest speedwells should be better regarded, for all-rounder status and for long-term, safe treatment of chronic but improvable conditions.

Try speedwell tea, distilled water or flower essence for yourself, and chances are you will experience similar sensations to those we had for the tincture.

It is as mentally clarifying as ground ivy tea but also feels nourishing in the body. The various speedwells we have tried have similar restorative effects, though with subtle differences eg slender speedwell lacks the grounding effect of germander speedwell.

In Ireland the plants were known as 'sore eyes', because an infusion was made into a lotion for tired eyes. At one time it shared the name 'eyebright' with *Euphrasia*, the better-known eyebright.

There is no reason why the tea cannot be used productively today for coughs or skin conditions, as it once was; similarly, a 'wound herb' does not lose its effectiveness just because it has gone out of fashion. Treben recommends speedwell compresses for *all inflamed, non-healing wounds*.

Interestingly, a Gaelic name for thyme-leaved speedwell translates as 'herb of the whooping cough', and modern research confirms that this plant contains scutellarin, a compound named from the calming herb skullcap.

The tea and other speedwell preparations can be considered whenever there is nervous exhaustion brought on by mental overload. Treben notes how two cups a day of equal amounts of horsetail and speedwell tea helped a priest remember the words in his sermons: he reportedly exclaimed: *my memory lapses disappeared surprisingly*.

Brooklime used to be eaten with watercress and oranges against scurvy. Modern forager John Wright doesn't much like the taste, but comes up with four reasons to write about brooklime: *it is edible, it's good for you, it's very common and the Latin name is fun*.

Thyme-leaved speedwell had a specific use for Native American Indians as a juice for earache, along with poultices for boils and a tea for chills and coughs.

Brooklime, a non-terrestrial speedwell, with fleshy edible leaves and stems

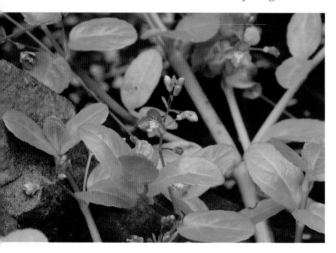

Germander speedwell is mainly used for itchy skin and as a wound herb, while heath speedwell, the 'official' medicinal herb, shares the uses of the other species.

Modern research
V. officinalis had anti-inflammatory effects on human lung cells on a molecular level, but has yet to be tested in clinical trials. It was found to be a deinhibitor of COX 2 (2013). Another study of V. officinalis (1985) showed anti-gastric ulcer activity in rats and regenerated mucosa, seeming to confirm popular observation.

V. ciliata, a plant used in Traditional Chinese Medicine, showed (2014) strong antioxidant properties on the liver and was protective for acute hepatoxicity, as a free-radical scavenger.

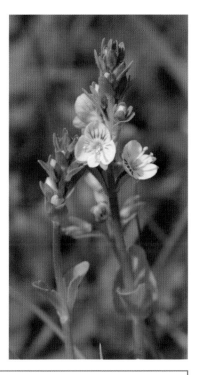

Thyme-leaved speedwell has tiny white flowers with delicate purple stripes

Speedwell tea
We usually choose germander speedwell, but use whichever species is common where you live. Put a few sprigs per person in a teapot and infuse in boiling water for about 20 minutes.

Speedwell foot bath
Use whichever species is common where you live – we have tried germander, field and ivy-leaved speedwells. Make a big pot of strong tea with your plants, then pour the plants and all into a basin large enough to put your feet in. Add warm water as necessary to top up. Soak your feet for about 20 minutes, adding new hot water if needed.

One of our students cycled home in record time after her speedwell foot bath, and said she felt energised all evening.

Germander speedwell flower essence
Follow the instructions for forget-me-not flower essence on page 75 to make your essence. Take a few drops on the tongue several times daily.

Speedwell tea
• restores
• energises

Speedwell foot bath
• restores
• energises
• refreshes tired feet

Germander speedwell flower essence
• clears the sight
• shifts awareness
• spiritual homesickness
• clarity of perception
• grounding

Sphagnum moss *Sphagnum* spp.

**Sphagnaceae
Sphagnum family**

Description: Dense colonies, with individuals up to 30cm (12in) high, with species varying from light green to red; branched, with stem leaves, inconspicuous flowers and brown, raised spore stalks.

Habitat: Peat bogs, a highly acidic, wet and anaerobic environment.

Distribution: Uplands of western and central Britain, especially Scotland and Ireland; northern Eurasia and North America, New Zealand, Chile.

Related species: The standard British and Irish field guide describes 34 species. These have similar medicinal and economic properties.

Parts used: Whole plant, dried and sorted.

[By using sphagnum] *Time and suffering are saved, as well as expense; the absorbent pads of moss are soft, elastic and very comfortable, easily packed and convenient to handle.*
– Grieve (1931)

Sphagnum moss (also peat or bog moss) has a spectacular capacity to absorb blood, is antiseptic, and easy to collect and transport. These properties made it a superb battlefield or foraging medicine; if you are cut while outdoors, yarrow or any astringent will stop bleeding and sphagnum can be the dressing.

Sphagnum moss is a denizen, and indeed creator, of peat bog habitats from tropics to poles, comprising some 120 species worldwide. In northern Eurasia and North America it was an early coloniser of the wasteland left by retreating ice caps. In effect it was a green bandage that healed the scars of the scourged frozen land under anaerobic pioneer vegetation that would become deep layers of peat.

The word 'bandage' is appropriate in human terms too, for sphagnum has been a wound dressing since prehistoric times; one Bronze Age warrior buried in Lothian had a chest wound packed with moss, while records of the Irish–Viking battle at Clontarf (1014) and the Scots–English encounter at Flodden (1513) refer to sphagnum dressings applied by field doctors.

Why is this plant so good as a natural bandage? The answer relates to sphagnum's structure. Its stem leaves consist of green or red photosynthetic cells and large, inert hyaline cells, which make up most of the plant's volume. The purpose of these dead cells is to absorb liquids and store them, which they do so well that some sphagnum species take in over 25 times their own weight in liquid.

A significant research finding is that pathogenic bacteria and human blood cells, as well as water, pass readily through sphagnum's hyaline cells. Hyaline cells have spiral thickening, which means they do not collapse if the moss dries out or is wrung out – that is, the moss is reusable.

Also the cell walls are rich in groups of pectic polysaccharides, known as sphagnan. These pectins ionise at low pH values (about 2, while the pH of blood is about 7.4). This means that sphagnum will lower the pH of its environment (ie acidify it) and inhibit pathogenic bacterial growth, which needs a more neutral-to-alkaline environment.

In practice, then, sphagnum will absorb astonishing quantities of water, blood, serum, pus and other liquids, while also being strongly antiseptic. In 1914–18 this made for a telling combination of life-supporting virtues in conditions

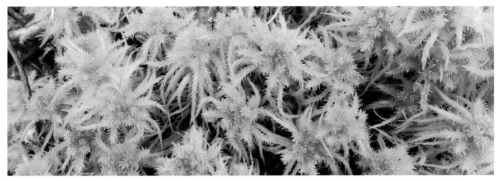

of trench warfare, where wounds easily suppurated and water soon became microbial-rich sewage.

Gathering of sphagnum for the British war effort owed much to an Edinburgh surgeon and RAMC lieutenant-colonel, Charles Walker Cathcart, who officially organised large-scale gathering, collection and forwarding to the battlefields.

Field surgeons found the moss superior to cotton wool for dressings: cotton was less absorbent, not antiseptic, less reusable and increasingly scarce as the war dragged on. Not only was the imported supply erratic but cotton was being diverted to the manufacture of explosives.

Meanwhile, crofters, girl guides and volunteers collected a cheap, endless supply of sphagnum from western Scotland and Dartmoor, and later Ireland. By 1918 one million dressings a month were sent to the trenches, including by then from Canada and the USA. One assistant in Edinburgh offered her thanks in verse (see right).

Garlic juice was routinely added to the sphagnum dressings as extra antiseptic. Many Allied lives were saved by such shrewd valuation of old herbal knowledge.

Other, civilian uses of sphagnum ought not to be forgotten: in various cultures, especially in Northern Europe, Canada and the Himalayas, it has made an easily gathered, free and soft material for nappies, menstrual pads and boot liners; it can stuff mattresses and pillows, and makes good insulation and animal bedding.

Solidified as peat, sphagnum was for long the traditional Irish fuel; New Zealand has a thriving trade in exporting the moss for hanging basket liners; it is used in potting soil mixes and is also a germination medium for orchids and fungi. It has been used to kill microbes and latterly to monitor air pollution.

Sphagnum is beautiful and eminently useful; it is, in the words of Simple Minds, a 'don't you (forget about me)' plant.

The doctors and the nurses
Look North with eager eyes,
And call on us to send them
The dressing that they prize.
No other is its equal –
In modest bulk it goes
Until it meets the gaping wound
Where the red life blood flows,
Then spreading, swelling in its might
It checks the fatal loss,
And kills the germ, and heals the hurt
– The kindly Sphagnum Moss.
– Mrs A M Smith, a member of the Edinburgh War Dressings Supply organisation, 1917

It is a good thing to know … when one is traveling in the wild, and needs to bandage a wound, because not only does the Sphagnum Moss act as an absorbent, but it seems to have antiseptic qualities. … one should not hesitate to use this moss.
– Coon (1957)

Sweet chestnut *Castanea sativa*

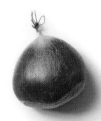

Fagaceae
Beech family

Description: Tall (to 30m, 100ft), deciduous tree, formerly coppiced; deeply fissured and twisted bark; longest leaves of any wild British tree (to 30cm, 1ft), deeply serrated, narrow, emerald green; long, beige male flower spikes and smaller green female flowers; sharply spiked cupules, each with 1 to 3 brown nuts with pointed ends.

Habitat: Usually planted in Britain, but self-propagates in south; nuts may not ripen in north.

Distribution: From Middle East, naturalised in Mediterranean and Northern Europe; also native to China, Japan; introduced to India, US, Australasia.

Related species: Not related to horse chestnut (*Aesculus hippocastanum*). *Castanea dentata* is the very tall (to 60m, 200ft) native North American species, decimated by blight in the first half of the 20th century, now being replanted; the Japanese sweet chestnut is *C. crenata*, and the Chinese form is *C. mollisima*.

Parts used: Leaves, nuts (fruit), buds.

Sweet chestnut is an ancient food crop of mountainous Mediterranean areas, the nuts often replacing grain as a source of flour. The leaves are a traditional medicinal treatment in respiratory conditions such as whooping cough and croup, for sore throat and diarrhoea, and the flowers are a Bach flower remedy. It is also in the news as a potential treatment for the 'superbug' MRSA that acts differently from antibiotics.

Sweet chestnut is an ancient food crop in the Mediterranean, being cultivated for over 4,000 years; older records exist for China, and in Japan it was used before rice.

The ground-up nuts are the source of an edible flour that has little protein or fat and no gluten, but twice as much starch as potato.

John Evelyn's pioneering book on trees, *Sylva* (1664), noted that *The bread of the flower* [flour] *is exceeding nutritive; 'tis a robust food, and makes women well complexion'd, as I have read.* He added the conventional wisdom that the nuts are liable to be windy, and could swell the belly and exacerbate colic.

But overall Evelyn was full of praise: the tree is *a magnificent and royal ornament* whose flour should be used by Britain's 'common people', rather than fed to pigs.

Sweet chestnut has long been used for animal fodder and litter, a timber and fuel, and the sweet Italian honey, *miele di castagno.*

Use sweet chestnut for...
Medicinally, says Thomas Bartram (1995), it is a *drying astringent, antirheumatic, antitussive.* It is best known for the last of these, as a leaf tea or tincture for dry and violent spasmodic coughs, such as whooping cough and croup, and as a gargle for sore throat.

Bartram suggests mixing 2 parts sweet chestnut and 1 part wild cherry bark for whooping cough. Pechey (1707) proposed a spoonful of the flour mixed with honey as 'a first-rate remedy' for coughs and 'spitting of blood'.

As a drying astringent the leaves and tincture remain effective for catarrh and diarrhoea. As an antirheumatic it has been found beneficial for muscular rheumatism, back pain and joints.

To complete its medicinal profile, sweet chestnut is one of the original 38 Bach Flower Remedies (taken to counteract despair and depression by faith and self-belief).

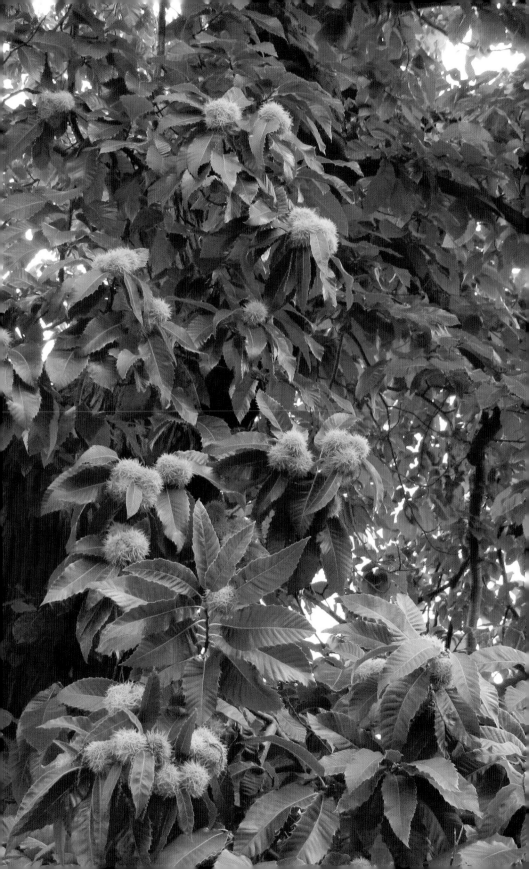

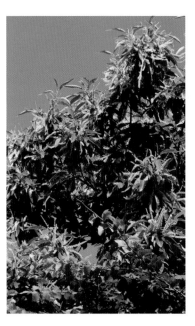

Sweet chestnut flowers, Norfolk, July

The study included the hospital 'superbug' MRSA (methicillin-resistant *Staphylococcus aureus*) as an SSTI, as it often presents as a skin infection.

Three herbs stood out powerfully: sweet chestnut, black horehound (*Ballota nigra*) and dwarf elder (*Sambucus ebulus*). A publication by Dr Quave and colleagues in August 2015 focused on sweet chestnut leaves, showing that ursene and oleanene derivatives (triterpenes) in the leaves inhibited quorum-sensing (QS) pathways, or cellular communication, in MRSA pathogens.

In conclusion, we have demonstrated that a folk-medical treatment [C. sativa] for skin inflammation and SSTIs that does not demonstrate 'typical' antibacterial activity (bacteriostatic or bactericidal) nevertheless shows great potential for development as a therapeutic due to its ability to specifically target and quench S. aureus virulence. The results of this study are important not only to future antibiotic discovery and development efforts, but are also vital to the validation of this previously poorly understood traditional medicine as an efficacious therapy, and not simply an unsubstantiated relict of folklore.
– Quave et al (2015)

The process involved the leaf extract shutting off the QS ability of the bacteria to create toxins that usually cause tissue damage. Dr Quave commented: *At the same time, the extract doesn't disturb the normal, healthy bacteria on human skin. It's all about restoring balance.* A single 50 microgram dose of the chestnut leaf extract cleared up MRSA skin lesions in mice, preventing further tissue and red blood cell damage. The extract did not lose activity, or become resistant, even after two weeks of repeated exposure.

The spring buds are a modern gemmotherapy treatment as a venous and lymphatic cleanser. Harvest the buds just before they open and extract in a mixture of alcohol, water and glycerine.

In rural southern Italy there is a current use of sweet chestnut leaves as a decoction for external treatment of skin infections, not found in British herblore.

Modern research
This empirically proven Italian method has been the focus of bioactive research by a team led by Dr Cassandra Quave of Atlanta's Emory University. The team tested over a hundred herbs used in Italian villagers' treatment of skin and soft tissue infections (SSTIs).

What is new here is that the 'disarming' of the communication channels of the pathogen offers an alternative to failing antibiotic methods that attempt to kill MRSA and eventually meet bacterial resistance. This is a significant step towards a post-antibiotic age.

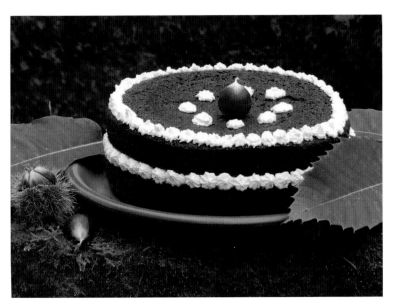

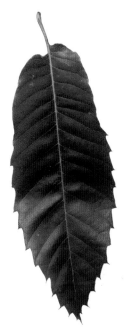

Sweet chestnut cake

John Pechey (right) would not approve, but we love this gluten-free cake, which can easily be vegan. Chestnut flour imparts a lovely flavour.

Preheat oven to 180°C. Sift into a large bowl: 2 cups **chestnut flour**, 1 cup **ground almonds**, ½ cup **cocoa powder**, 2 cups **light brown sugar**, 2 teaspoons **bicarbonate of soda**, 1 teaspoon **salt** and 3 tablespoons **linseed**, ground. Add 2 cups **water**, 2 tablespoons **vinegar**, 2 teaspoons **vanilla extract** and ½ cup melted **butter or coconut oil**.

Pour into two greased and floured 8-inch (20cm) round cake tins, and bake for 40 minutes, until a straw poked into the centre comes out clean. Cool, then chill in the refrigerator before removing carefully from the tins. Layer together with **whipped cream** or **coconut cream**.

Antibacterial ointment

Chop up a handful of **sweet chestnut leaves** and place in a small saucepan with enough **extra virgin olive oil** to cover. Heat gently for half an hour, then strain out the leaves, measure the oil and return to the pan.

Add 10g **beeswax** for every 100ml of oil. Heat and stir until the wax has melted, then pour the ointment into jars.

In some Places beyond Sea they make Bread and Frumenty of the Flower [flour] of the Nuts; but such sort of course Diet is in no way pleasing to the English, who (God be thanked) have Plenty of wholsom Food, and great Abundance of all things necessary.
– Pechey (1707)

Antibacterial ointment
- cuts
- grazes
- pimples
- boils
- skin infections

Thistle *Cirsium* spp.

Milk and blessed thistle are commercial-scale medicinal herbs, but other wild species, such as spear/bull, creeping/Canada and marsh thistle, have a traditional and potential healing reputation. Thistle's alkalinity in medicinal drinks and for treatment of joints and arthritis are exciting prospects.

Asteraceae
Daisy family

Description: Spiny biennials/perennials; with pink, purple or yellow flowerheads; often tall and erect; spear thistle (*Cirsium vulgare*) is downy, with single pink flowers, winged leaves; creeping thistle (*C. arvense*) has scented lilac flowers; marsh thistle (*C. palustre*) is reedy, with clustered flowers.

Habitat: Waste ground, hedgerows, waysides, fields; marsh thistle needs dampness.

Distribution: Widespread in Europe, Western Asia; naturalised in North America, Australasia, often termed invasive/noxious weeds.

Related species: Milk thistle (*Silybum marianum*) and blessed thistle (*Cnicus benedictus*) are commercial medicinals; others, eg musk (*Carduus nutans*), dwarf (*Cirsium acaule*), welted (*Carduus crispus*) and slender thistle (*Carduus tenuiflorus*), are similar medicinally.

Parts used: Roots, leaves, stems, flowers.

The thistle is the quintessential Scottish emblem, but 'Scotch thistle' is not native to Scotland – it is actually the cotton thistle (*Onopordum acanthium*), a white downy thistle from East Anglia.

We can even pin a date on the arrival of the symbolic Scotch thistle to its 'homeland'. It was the novelist Sir Walter Scott who, in 1822, masterminded the visit of George IV to Scotland, and quickly invented several 'traditions' for the monarch's pleasure, including restoring banned tartans/clans, and choosing a national thistle.

Oddly, there is a thistle that occurs almost wholly in Scotland – the melancholy thistle (*Cirsium heterophyllum*). But it is literally spineless, has soft flowers and is pretty rather than formidable – not at all apt for Scott's purposes.

If you want a wild native thistle for Scotland, or for any other part of the British Isles, look to spear thistle (*Cirsium vulgare*), creeping or field thistle (*C. arvense*) and marsh thistle (*C. palustre*). These are widespread members of the Cardueae subgroup of non-latex-producing thistles, with burdocks, milk thistle, globe artichoke, knapweeds and cotton thistle.

For the record, the other subgroup of the true thistles is the Lactuceae, which do yield latex. Among these species are chicory, the lettuces, nippleworts, hawkbits, oxtongues, sowthistles, dandelions and mouse-ear hawkweeds.

Spines and latex are of course defensive mechanisms for thistles, making them unpalatable to animal browsers. For, as forager Miles Irving notes, if you have formidable defensive weapons like these you don't need additional bitterness as a deterrent.

This is why wild thistles make a good, sweet food source. This is additional to the cultivated eating thistles like artichoke and cardoon. So thistle roots, stalks, peeled stems and basal leaves are all targets for the forager, as they were in subsistence times before.

There are no poisonous thistles, for much the same reason, and

Spear or bull thistle,
Cirsium vulgare

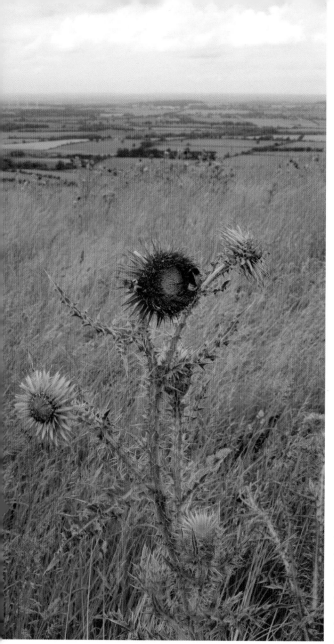

But these symbolic, edible plants also have a disreputable side in British farming. Spear thistle and creeping thistle are defined as injurious weeds under the Weeds Act 1959. This means that farmers must take steps to prevent their spread (along with three other plants: curled dock, broad-leaved dock and common ragwort).

Spear thistle is known as bull thistle in North America, and is noxious in nine US states. It has a similar status in Australia. Creeping thistle is called Canada thistle in the US, but is actually the imported European plant.

Use thistle for...
Milk thistle (*Silybum marianum*) and blessed thistle (*Cnicus benedictus*) are well-known and cultivated as herbal remedies, and can be found in any good herbal.

In 1812 Sir John Hill could state that milk thistle was *a very beautiful plant, common by roadsides*. Both thistles can still be found wild in the British Isles but now in insufficient abundance to consider them true 'wayside plants' and be included here.

Broadly speaking, the wild thistles share the hepatoprotective (liver-supporting) and cholagogue (bile-secreting) properties of the mainstream, cultivated thistles, but with lesser strength of action.

Milk thistle has the highest percentage of silibinin flavonoids,

Musk thistle, *Carduus nutans*, White Horse Hill, Uffington, Oxfordshire, August

indeed thistles will counteract strong poisons, including some fungi. The main downside for foragers, apart from getting behind the barrage of spines, is that perennial thistles, eg creeping thistle, become woody and tough.

which are the active constituent of the standardised extract silymarin. This is antioxidant, blocks damaging toxins in the liver and stimulates liver cell growth.

Silymarin is widely used in pharmaceutical products for liver cirrhosis, chronic hepatitis and prostate cancer treatment.

Spear thistle has an older reputation in cancer treatments, and as a cardiac tonic. In this light, herbalist Julian Barker suggests that cotton thistle *is perhaps deserving of the kind of investigation that Globe Artichoke has received.*

Creeping or Canada thistle was a leaf tea 'tonic' and diuretic, once used for treating tuberculosis internally and for skin eruptions, ulcers and poison ivy rash externally. Its root tea was for dysentery and diarrhoea. Another old country remedy, found in Scotland and various parts of England, was for a thistle tea for depression (as was melancholy thistle) or chronic headaches.

An altogether more modern take on thistle drinks is that of American herbalist Katrina Blair. She focuses on the alkalinity of thistle, as a juice or made into a chai, lemonade or tea.

Blair reminds us that almost all disease arises from over-acidity in the body. Modern life adds to this acidity via pollution, pesticides and preservatives, refined foods and stress, among other toxic factors, but thistles can readily supply bioavailable alkalinity.

Julie can add another idea for improving alkalinity: regular deep breathing raises pH levels towards 7, the alkalinity threshold.

Modern research
There is a fascinating finding by American herbalist Matthew Alfs (2014) regarding potential use of bull (spear) thistle (*Cirsium vulgare*) tincture in treating spondyloarthropathy (SpA).

Alfs says clinical trials appear *to confirm a little-known, folk-medicinal tradition that* C. vulgare *supports the health of joints, tendons and ligaments in a most remarkable way.* Treatment was based on a tincture

[For] *A Chronical Head-Ach: … take a large Tea-cup full of Carduus Tea, without Sugar, fasting for six or seven Mornings: Tried.* – Wesley (1765)

[For] *The Stone in the Kidneys: boil an Ounce of Thistle-root and four Drams of Liquorice in a Pint of Water. Drink half of it at a Time fasting.* – Wesley (1765)

Thistle stalks are a great source of mineralized, … highly alkanized water, … alive with the brilliance of the thistle plant. … Thistle offers the body a true alkaline experience. – Blair (2014)

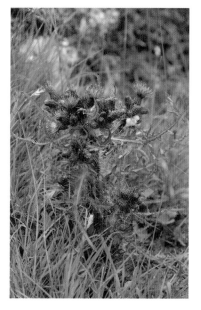

Marsh thistle, *Cirsium palustre*

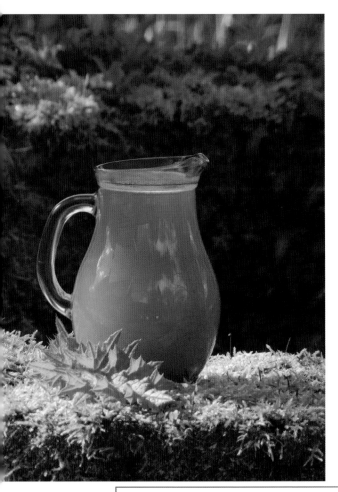

(100 proof vodka, ie 50% alcohol in UK terms), of first-year basal leaves, extracting for two to three weeks. The dosage was 6–10 drops per 20 lb of body weight, two to three times a day. Symptom relief and structural improvement were rapid, and were confirmed by medical doctors.

The mechanism appears to be bull thistle's action as a powerful anti-inflammatory, based on Native American oral traditions. The presence in bull thistle of the flavonoid genkwanin-4'O-glucoside (the only thistle to have it) may help the body's immune system identify and eliminate dormant bacteria.

The reports are promising for sufferers of juvenile SpA and some forms of arthritis caused by micro-organisms (hence not osteoarthritis, which is the result of joint overuse). Further trials will hopefully be undertaken.

Julie finds in her practice that a spear thistle tincture is helping patients who have Lyme disease with joint symptoms.

Green thistle energiser
- arthritis
- acidity
- liver health
- vitality

With thanks to Katrina Blair for inspiring this recipe

Green thistle energiser
We use spear thistle in this recipe, as it is the thistle we are fortunate (yes!) to have in our garden. It is biennial, so this drink is best made from the first-year rosette of leaves, before the thistle flowers in its second year. Cut at the base of the leaves where there are no spines.

Put in a blender: about 8 **thistle leaves** (or a whole thistle including roots if you are weeding), half an **unpeeled lemon**, and a 750ml bottle of **apple juice**. Blend until bright green. Strain the pulp out (gets rid of any spines), and drink the bright green liquid. This lemonade is delicious!

Valerian *Valeriana officinalis*

Valerian has been a useful food, perfume and medicine for over two thousand years, but with unexpected twists in its story. It has well-attested sedative and relaxant effects, but in some 'hot' patients can over-stimulate instead. Despite modern reservations on its root odour it is a valuable and effective herbal ally.

Wild valerian is a beautiful marsh and dryland plant, but its reputation is inseparable from its smell. The white-pink flowers have a vanilla-like odour that is delicate in single flowers and heady in colonies, while the smell of the roots is often dismissed in terms approaching disgust.

It would surprise our ancestors to read modern herbal accounts that describe dried valerian root as smelling like tom cats or old socks, as nauseating and unpleasant. An old Greek term *phu*, still applied in the name of some varieties of valerian, is sometimes said to be onomatopoeic, describing the sound of rejection (*phew!*) when encountering the roots.

This claim tells us much about a modern Western sensibility. In the past, valerian was thought to be sweet-smelling enough to place the roots among bedlinen, and a Japanese form of *Valeriana officinalis*, called kesso root, is a popular perfume, as is the related Indian valerian (*V. jatamansi*).

In modern commerce the oil of valerian is used in blended

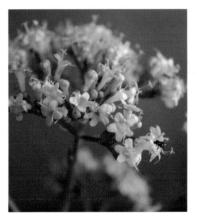

perfume oils, for 'mossy' and 'leathery' tones. Valerian essential oil in aromatherapy provides indications that its odour alone can have a sedative effect.

In addition to various medicinal uses, valerian leaves were a salad herb of the Anglo-Saxons. Gerard in 1597 related that valerian (or setwall, in another older name) was indispensable in *broths, pottage or physicall meats*.

A close relative is common cornsalad or lamb's lettuce (*Valerianella locusta*), a salad crop in our garden; it is locally wild in southern Britain and the US.

Caprifoliaceae Honeysuckle family

Description: Tall, perennial, to 2m (6ft), with sparse, erect stems and Apiaceae-like umbels of white-pink small, scented flowers; leaflets opposite; roots, rhizomes and stolons, highly scented when dried.

Habitat: Widespread in marshy land in Britain but also in limestone grassland (it was once grown commercially in Derbyshire).

Distribution: Widespread in Britain and Ireland. Introduced in Canada and northern US.

Related species: Marsh valerian (*V. dioica*) is rare and non-medicinal; red valerian (*Centranthus ruber*) is common in southern Britain, but also non-medicinal. Common cornsalad (*Valerianella locusta*) is another relative, which grows wild on thin poor soils, and makes a garden salad vegetable. Over 150 species worldwide; native in temperate Western Europe, Western Asia, USA.

Parts used: Roots, above-ground parts.

Valerian roots: this dense mat is the usual source of medicinals, though we like to use the flowers.

Cats find the smell of valerian hard to resist, with old stories of them breaking into apothecary shops to get to it. Valerian was once a rat bait, and some say the Pied Piper of Hamelin attracted the town's rodents more by hidden valerian root in his pockets than his hypnotic flute-playing!

Away from the smell and taste of valerian, its history reveals an interesting case of one individual

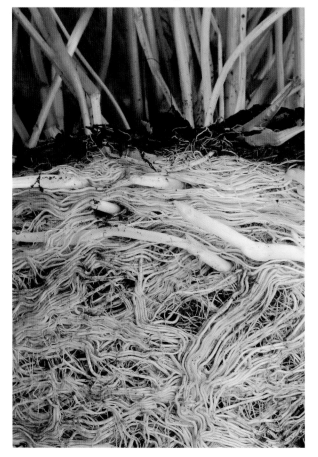

adapting a classic use of a plant for his personal health, thereby moving valerian to modern status.

Fabius Columna, or Fabio Colonna (1567–1650), was an early Italian plantsman, now largely forgotten. Born in Naples, he trained as a lawyer and linguist, but became interested in plants because from birth he had suffered from epilepsy and could not find a cure.

Contemporary physicians failing him, Columna went back fifteen hundred years to the source of European herbalism, Dioscorides. His *De Materia Medica* proposed valerian for similar purposes.

Columna dried valerian roots and swallowed the powder in various combinations of wine, water and milk. It was successful for him (though he may have relapsed later) and relieved symptoms in other people he treated too. Columna's *Phytobasanos* of 1592 publicised his experiences with valerian – and incidentally gave the world the flower term 'petal'.

The book made little impact in England, with the leading herbalists Gerard and Parkinson ignoring the epilepsy finding. John Pechey (1707), however, reported that Columna's use of valerian for epilepsy was *more effectual in this Case than the Roots of Male-Peony* [Paeonia mascula].

Columna's rediscovery of an ancient use for valerian opened

out its applications in treating nervous disorders more generally. By 1772 John Hill had published the 12th edition of his own book *The Virtue of Wild Valerian in Nervous Disorders*.

American herbalists of the 18th and 19th centuries helped bring valerian into mainstream medicine. It was included in the *U.S. Pharmacopoeia* as an anti-spasmodic and sleep aid from 1820 to 1936. Valerian remains 'official' as a sedative in the latest *British Herbal Pharmacopoeia* (1996).

But the smell issue was always there. The notorious tincture of valerian, Tincturea Valerianae ammoniata, mixing valerian root oil with oil of nutmeg and lemon, and ammonia, was described by Mrs Grieve (1931) as *an extremely nauseous and offensive preparation.*

Nonetheless it was a widely prescribed Victorian medicine. One example is Gustave Flaubert's novel, *Madame Bovary* (1856), where the country doctor Charles Bovary administers valerian to his fretful wife, Emma, for her nerves, along with camphor baths.

The tincture was used for shell-shock (now called post-traumatic stress disorder) in World War I and for treating civilians.

Finally, a word about **Red valerian** (*Centranthus ruber*), also known by a variety of attractive names like drunken sailor, bouncing Bess, pretty Betsy, kiss me quick, red money and scarlet lightning.

This member of the wider Valerian family was first recorded in Gerard's London garden in 1597. A fashionable introduction from Italy, he called it a 'great ornament' in his garden. It later spread around the west and south of England, and blows bright red in the wind from its haunts on city buildings. It has no medicinal uses, though the fleshy leaves are tender enough for spring salads.

… whereupon it hath been had (and is to this day among the poore people of our Northerne parts) in such veneration amongst them, that no broths, pottage or physicall meats are worth any thing, if Setwall [valerian] were not at an end.
– Gerard (1597)

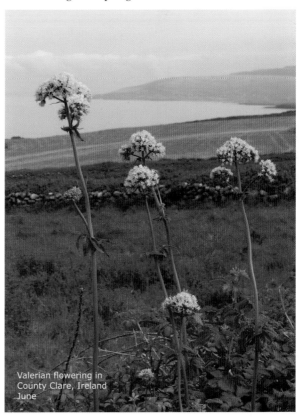
Valerian flowering in County Clare, Ireland
June

Use valerian for...

The medieval accolade 'all-heal' was conferred on valerian, and this name could be an English version of Latin *valere*, to be well. Indeed, the plant was known to Parkinson (1640) as a standby for headaches, colds and coughs, eye problems, colic and modest wound-healing (another old name for it was 'cut finger').

It is worth remembering these more mundane properties of valerian, which remain useful alongside its proven value as a sedative and relaxant for stress and tensions, whether musculoskeletal or nervous.

The American herbalist 7Song makes a pertinent point on people's reactions to the plant as a sedative. He finds, and others have confirmed, that about one in nine or ten people become agitated, 'wired' rather than calmed by it. Indeed he says this reaction is the most common contrary effect of any herb he uses.

He has adopted a conservative protocol for valerian. He will see a new insomnia patient around the middle of the day, in his office, and give them a small amount of fresh root valerian tincture as an initial test for their reaction. Dosage and treatment details are adjusted in light of the patient's response.

Julie finds valerian well indicated when stress or headache is accompanied by digestive problems; the tincture, tea or capsules can help reduce anxiety and panic attacks, palpitations and high blood pressure. Valerian has proven efficacy for insomnia accompanied by worries, fears and high emotion.

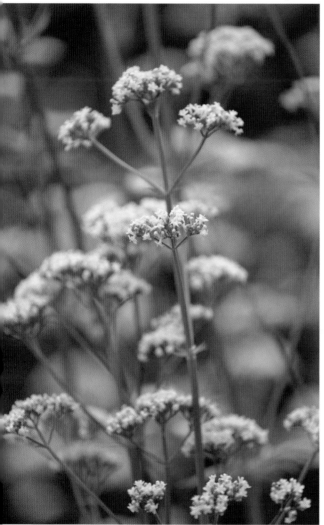

Above-ground parts of valerian: an under-used resource

As an antispasmodic valerian eases muscles of the stomach, shoulders and neck; the tightness of period pain and irritable bowel syndrome are also relieved.

Valerian combines well with other sedative and hypnotic remedies, like passionflower, hops, lemon balm and chamomile. It is best avoided when a patient is taking hypotensive medication, which can lead some to next-morning drowsiness, in which case drivers and users of heavy machinery should avoid the plant or the drug.

We think the above-ground parts should be used more, with milder but similar results for the patient. Baths, steam distillation and home flower essences are routes for further exploration. There are also commercial flower essences, including one for the nervous system and one for delight and joy.

Modern research
The pharmacology of valerian is complex, with over 150 compounds named already. Previous research efforts to identify specific compounds as causative, eg valepotriates or valeric acid, have latterly been displaced by emphasis on the synergistic positive actions of the plant as a whole. Or, use the herb!

Responses to valerian, as we have seen, can be paradoxical, and moreover its actions can vary, by locality (compare taller marshy plants with shorter limestone ones), seasonality, dosage, length of treatment (in case of cumulative effect) and preparation.

Such variations aside, valerian is in general safe, non-addictive (an important factor in sedatives) and effective as a dose-dependent herb for sleep-promotion.

Half a Spoonful of the Powder of the Root, before the Stalk springs, taken once or twice, in Wine, Water or Milk, relieves those that are seiz'd with the Falling-sickness [epilepsy].
– Pechey (1707)

Providing the dose is appropriate and the preparation is properly made and conserved from good quality plant material, Valerian is unquestionably the supreme remedy in all cases of nervous trouble either on its own or combined with other plants.
– Barker (2001)

Harvesting valerian
Traditionally, the roots of valerian are used, but we have found that the flowers also give good results. The flowers have a vanilla scent, but the tincture or glycerite has the same smell as the roots, which cats and some people love and others dislike. Our friend Glennie Kindred gave us a good tip for harvesting valerian root – grow it in a large pot sunk into the ground, then at the end of the summer lift the plant and harvest the roots that have been going round the inside of the pot. These can easily be trimmed, and the plant replanted with no ill effects.

Valerian flower glycerite
Pick enough **valerian flowers** to fill a jar. Add 4 parts **vegetable glycerine** and 1 part **vodka** to cover the flowers. Leave in a warm sunny place for 2 to 4 weeks, strain out and bottle the liquid.

Dosage: Take a teaspoonful before bed for help with sleep, or ½ teaspoon several times daily for anxiety.

Valerian flower glycerite
• insomnia
• anxiety
• digestive tension
• tension headache
• neck & shoulder tension

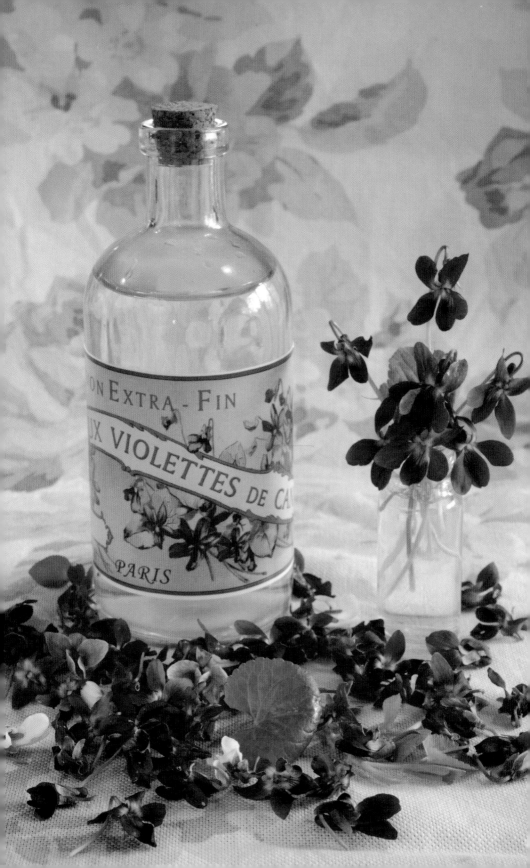

Violet *Viola odorata*

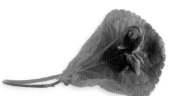

Sweet violets have always been valued for their beauty and scent, and as a syrup, crystallised sweet or a tea they are on the pleasant and child-friendly side of medicinal. They nonetheless act powerfully as expectorants for the respiratory tract, as cooling for hot and inflammatory conditions, particularly of the skin, and as an ally in some forms of cancer treatment.

Sweet violets have long been celebrated for their perfume and springtime beauty, peeping up in shady woods when the snowdrops finish. Dog violet species are later-flowering but equally beautiful, the rather disparaging 'dog' in their name referring to their lack of scent (in the same way as the unscented wild rose is a dog rose).

An early Western herbal, written by Macer in the 12th century, sets out the conventional valuation of violets: *Neither the rose colour ne the lylie may over-passe the violet, neither in beaute, neither in strengthe or vertue, neither in odour.*

Among the many poets who couldn't get enough of them was the Romantic Leigh Hunt, who in 1820 coined the phrase 'shrinking violet', for the plant's apparent modesty. He clearly wasn't aware that the carpet of purple violets he admired was the result of its vigorous and competitive runners.

A much earlier poet, Horace (65–8 BC), lamented that his fellow Romans spent more time growing violets to flavour their wine than growing olives. As the ancients knew, violets lend their colour and scent to liquids – wine, water (teas), syrup, vinegar or honey.

Violet flowers are cooling and demulcent, and had a reputation among the Greeks and Romans as a remedy for easing drunkenness and headaches, when applied to the head as a garland. Richard Surflet, in 1600, repeated the formula: *The flowers of March violets applied unto the brows, doe assuage the headach, which commeth of too much drinking and procure sleepe.*

Violets were also much used for the complexion – think of the Victorian obsession with violet water. Earlier, the Rev John Lightfoot, writing in 1777 of Scottish customs, advised his female readers irresistibly: *Anoint thy face with goat's milk in which violets have been infused and there is not a young prince on earth who would not be charmed with thy beauty.*

Violaceae
Violet family

Description: Sweet violet (*Viola odorata*), named for its scent, spreads largely by runners; has early spring flowers, usually purple but can be white or pink-red, and heart-shaped leaves.

Habitat: Usually lowlands in British Isles (except mountain pansy, *V. lutea*), woods with light shade, roadsides, hedgebanks; prefer lime-rich soils (except marsh violet, *V. palustris*); pansies favour arable fields with disturbed ground.

Distribution: Europe, North America, India and China; also many garden species, which hybridise with wild violets or are escapes.

Related species: About 20 British Violas, notably common dog violet (*V. riviniana*); of the pansies field pansy (*V. arvensis*) is more abundant than heartsease, wild pansy (*V. tricolor*); in North America Canada violet (*V. canadensis*) is widespread, as is common blue violet (*V. sororia*). All Viola species can be used medicinally.

Parts used: Flowers, leaves, root.

Etching of sweet violet and associated insects by Maria Sibylla Merian (1717), John Innes Historical Collections, courtesy of the John Innes Foundation

One 'young prince' we know well is Shakespeare's Hamlet. In an early scene of the play Laertes warns his sister Ophelia about Hamlet's volatile temperament. Sweet violet's smell is the chosen apt metaphor: *A violet in the youth of primy nature, / Forward, not permanent, sweet, not lasting, / The perfume and suppliance of a minute. / No more.*

What perfumiers (and dramatists) long knew pharmacologists confirm: compounds from violets called ionones have been isolated,

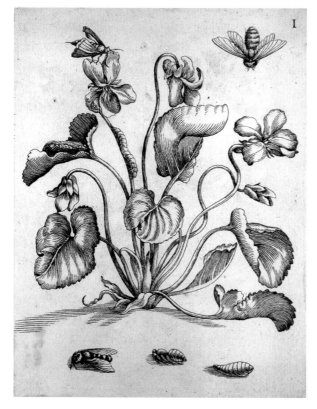

which temporarily block our sense of smell, then release it. This means violets smell good to us over and over again – perhaps the secret of their enduring appeal?

It is not only the flowers that go into perfume. The famous Vera Violetta perfume (1892) used sweet violet leaves. Most violet perfume today, regrettably, is synthetic.

Use violets for...
The violet group (Violas) broadly consists of violets and pansies, including heartsease, but we are focused on true violets here. Heartsease is useful for heart concerns, skin problems such as eczema, lymphatic congestion, bladder irritation and cancer.

Behind violet's idealised image lies a coarser truth: it makes you spit. That is, violets are technically expectorants, and are still 'official' in Britain for this use. One area of their action is described as pectoral, for relieving chest issues such as harsh coughs, asthma, whooping cough and bronchitis.

The plant also contains mucilage, contributing to a demulcent effect of soothing an irritated respiratory tract, stomach or intestines. Violet is also used by herbalists for its anti-tumour action, especially for breast, lung and gastrointestinal cancers.

Violet syrup is a traditional and still-used remedy for children suffering from coughs and croup, with the additional benefit of lowering cough-related fevers. The syrup acts as a gentle juvenile laxative and was also used as a mouthwash for inflamed gums and a gargle for sore throats.

Violet's cooling properties as a tea or syrup come into play where there is excess heat or inflammation, including migraines with feelings of heat, and for arthritis and rheumatism. Externally, violet poultices will reduce the pain of swellings or cracked nipples, and ease inflammatory skin issues, such as eczema, psoriasis and acne, and cradle cap in babies.

The root of violet was once used as a purgative – much more 'medicinal' than the syrup, and stretching Culpeper's view of violet to its limit: … *a fine pleasing*

plant of Venus, of a mild nature and no way hurtful.

In cases when sickness prevents sleep, Askham's herbal (1550) recommended boiling violet plants in water and soaking the feet 'to the ancles'; when the patient goes to bed, the herb should be bound to his temples, *and he shall slepe wel, by the grace of God.*

American herb scientist James Duke suggests eating violet flowers can help treat varicose and spider veins. He reasons that the flowers contain generous amounts of rutin, which supports capillary wall integrity and strength.

An infusion made of violet leaves eases tension headaches and was a reputable cancer remedy from medieval times. Among South Africa's black population in the 1980s violet leaves were chewed

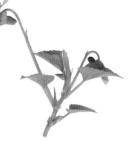

Dog violet

To dispel drunkenness and repel migraine/ The violet is sovereign;/ From heavy head it takes the pain,/ And from feverish cold delivers the brain.
– Regimen Sanitatis Salernitanum (*The Salernitan Rule of Health*), c. 12thc.

The decoction of Violets is good against all hote Fevers, and all inward inflammations, … The syrupe is good against the inflammations of the lungs and breast, the pleurisie and cough, and also against fevers, especially in children.
– Langham (1583)

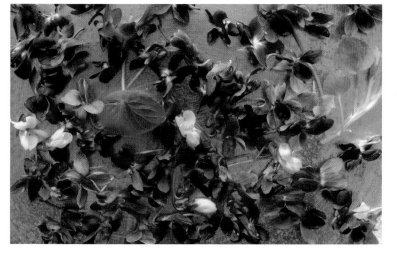

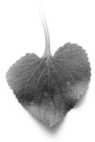

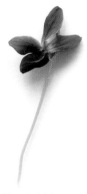

Violet leaf tea
• sore throats
• coughs
• inflammation
• mild constipation

Violet glycerite
• mild asthma
• sore throats
• coughs
• inflammation
• mild constipation

and also crushed to make a poultice applied to skin cancers and abnormal skin growths. This 'neoplastic' quality of violet now attracts clinical research, as does its potential value in breast and stomach cancer treatment, HIV and immune disorders.

Modern research
The Viola family is rich in novel plant-protective peptides called cyclotides, and 1995 research identified cycloviolacin O1.

A study into cycloviolacins in *Viola odorata* (2010a) found them to be promising chemosensitising agents against drug-resistant breast cancer; a similar study of the same compounds in *V. tricolor* (2010b) showed them to be cytotoxic in cancer cell lines.

The same cyclotides were isolated in Chinese medicinal herb *V. yedoensis* (*zi hua di ding*) (2008), and showed anti-HIV activity through disrupting HIV cell membranes. Another Chinese study (2011) found the same plant antibacterial to various forms of *Streptococcus* and to *E. coli* and *Salmonella* through its coumarin content.

Confirming traditional uses, Iranian research (2014) found an essential oil from *Viola odorata* (two drops taken nasally before sleep) offered relief to 50 patients with chronic insomnia.

A study (2015) of sweet violet, via a flower syrup was used in a double-blind randomised controlled trial to treat 182 children with intermittent asthma.

Harvesting violets
Because sweet violet spreads mainly by runners rather than seed in spring (if there is a second flowering in autumn, the reverse is true), your picking of the flowers will not affect its viability. It also grows in colonies, but only pick what you need.

The leaves can be picked year round in milder areas, but are at their best in spring and summer. They can readily be dried for use throughout the year.

Violet leaf tea
Use 2 or 3 fresh **leaves** or a rounded teaspoon of crumbled dried leaves per mug of **boiling water**. Leave to infuse for at least 5 minutes, then strain and drink.

Violet flower glycerite
Fill a small jar with **sweet violet flowers**, then pour in **vegetable glycerine** to fill. Shake and keep the jar in a warm place until the violets lose their colour, then strain and bottle.

Crystallised violets

The crystallising liquid used in this vegan recipe is best prepared ahead of time, as the gum arabic can take some time to dissolve.

Put in a small jar: 1 tablespoon **gum arabic powder** (also called Acacia gum) with 3 tablespoons **water or rosewater**. Shake well and leave overnight for the powder to dissolve. This mixture will keep in the fridge for months.

Pick about 20 **violets**, leaving some stalk on each flower. Dip a flower into the liquid, holding it by the stem. Shake off as much excess liquid as you can, then sprinkle the flower with **caster (superfine) sugar** and hang it on the edge of a cup or glass to dry – the stem has a handy bend that makes this easy. Once the cup rim is full, you can put it in an airing cupboard to speed drying, or the violets can be laid gently on a dehydrator tray to finish drying.

When the violets are dry, keep them in an airtight jar until you want to use them. Unlike violets that have been crystallised with egg white, these will keep for a year or more as long as they are stored airtight.

Sweet violets

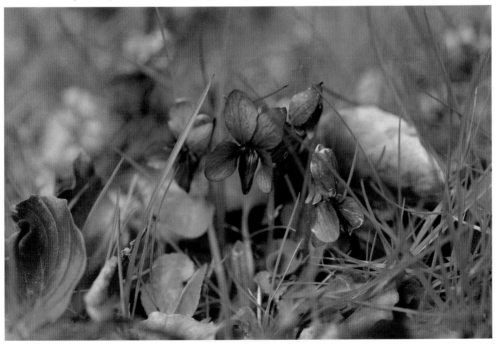

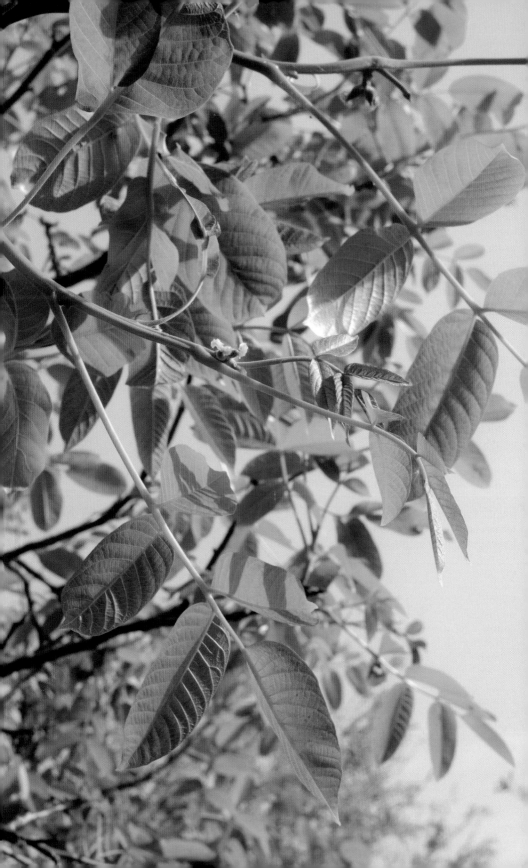

Walnut *Juglans regia*

Juglandaceae
Walnut family

Description: A graceful tree growing to 25m (80ft); lime-green oval leaves with 3 to 9 leaflets, aromatic but with a smell coarsening as leaves mature and dry; soft green husks harden into a shell, turning the familar beige brown; flesh is in two 'brain-like', nutritious halves.

Habitat: Likes temperate conditions but grows to 2,000m (7,000ft) altitude; sensitive to late frosts.

Distribution: Native to central Asia, introduced across Northern Hemisphere.

Related species: Black walnut (*Juglans nigra*) and butternut (white walnut) (*J. cinerea*) in North America, and paper-shell walnut (*J. mandschurica*) in China. Pecans and hickories are closely related North American nuts.

Parts used: Bark, leaves, husks, green and ripe nuts.

Walnut was thought by the Romans and Greeks to be native to Persia (Iran), from where it spread by trade both to the west and east in ancient times. Central Asia is now regarded as the likely origin. The nut, both green and brown, and leaves are the main parts used, and the tree enjoys an enviable reputation as a food, aphrodisiac, wood, oil, dye and medicine.

The scientific names of the common walnut recall an elite, even a divine past: *Juglans* meant 'nuts of Jupiter' and *regia* was royal. A 'food of the gods' to the Romans meant that walnuts conferred sexual vigour, and who was more vigorous than the god Jupiter? Among common mortals walnuts were symbolically thrown at Roman weddings.

We now know that walnuts contain plentiful arginine and zinc, both of which support the human sexual response. In more general terms eating walnuts regularly has long been known as good practice for maintaining vigorous health, especially in older age.

Walnuts have been a **food** from prehistoric times and across every culture where the tree grows. The nuts are light in weight and a handy size to gather and carry, and are highly nutritious.

In current terminology walnuts are a superfood that can reduce cholesterol levels and have a positive effect on heart health.

Walnuts have high levels of polyunsaturates, especially omega-3 fatty acids, which is good news for health but unfortunately not for the nut's storage. Even with modern freezing methods walnuts remain prone to rancidity.

The green, unripe rinds are edible, if sour, as well as being good for pickling. John Parkinson (1640) wrote that preserved green nuts in sugar made a 'dainty junket', and also good for 'weake stomackes'.

As a **wood**, walnut was the English cabinet-maker's timber of choice until imported mahogany largely supplanted it in the 18th century, though it remains popular. It proved unsuitable for house- or ship-building, however.

Walnut oil is used for salads and for cooking in southern Europe, but is costly, partly because it does not keep well. It also has too low a boiling point for good frying.

American black walnut in particular yields an excellent fast **dye**. A black stain emerges

Why Wall-Nuts, having no affinity with a wall [should be so called]. The truth is, Gual or Wall to the Old Dutch signifieth 'strange' or 'exotick' (whence Welsh, that is foreigners); these nuts being no natives of England or Europe, and probably first fetch'd from Persia.
– Fuller (1682)

... in several places twixt Hanaw and Francfort in Germany, no young farmer whatsoever is permitted to marry a wife, till he bring proof that he hath planted, and is a father of such a stated number of walnut-trees, as the law is inviolably observed to this day, for the extraordinary benefit which this tree affords the inhabitants.
– Evelyn (1664)

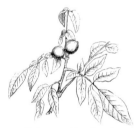

Walnut, etching by JC Loudon (1838)

I felt moved and elated by the universally cordial atmosphere that suffused the forest [ie the walnut forests of Kyrgyzstan] ... Everyone gave us walnuts, always choosing their very best. Our pockets swelled, our hands blackened.
– Deakin (2007)

easily from the nuts, both in green and ripe stages, and handling is inevitably messy – users beware!

The mature nut, as everybody knows, resembles the **human brain** in miniature (in Afghanistan the nut is called *charmarghz*, or 'four brains'). Herbalist William Coles, writing in 1657, said the nuts had 'the perfect Signature of the Head', meaning that walnuts resembled a brain so must be useful for brain treatment. And he just might be proved right.

Use walnut for...
Walnut species in the temperate world have similar medicinal actions, with common astringent, tonic and anti-inflammatory properties, among others.

Native Americans, for example, had a range of uses for black walnut (and later the settler-introduced common walnut): as an expectorant and purgative; to treat toothache, headache and greying hair; for colic, diarrhoea and skin complaints; as an insecticide and antifungal.

In early modern Europe walnut was a pestilence or plague herb. Culpeper, for one, stated of the green unripe nuts: *you shall find them exceeding comfortable to the stomach, they resist poison, and are a most excellent preservative against the Plague, inferior to none.*

In London's plague year of 1666, the eminent doctor Thomas

Willis offered *For the Poorer Sort, that Recipe of the Ancients*. This was two handfuls of rue, fig and walnut kernels (24 each), and half an ounce of salt, all beaten in a mortar. Parkinson in 1640 had attributed a similar plague recipe to Mithridates, king of Pontus (135–63 BC).

The action the apothecaries and physicians were looking for here was in the expectorant, emetic and purgative spectrum. Dried and powdered walnut bark taken as a tea could produce any of these responses, depending on dosage.

The green, unripe shell and the early green leaves have high astringency, utilised widely as a gargle for mouth and throat ulcers. In mild doses an infusion of green walnuts would soothe coughs, asthma and stomach ulcers, while stronger doses were for dissolving stones and cancerous tumours.

Other well-established uses included walnut as a blackening hair dye, though the Roman naturalist Pliny's two thousand-year-old recipe will be less popular now: boil green walnut husks with lead, ashes, oil and earthworms, and paste on the head.

Externally, cooled walnut tea was applied to inflammatory skin conditions such as eczema and herpes simplex via rubbing, compresses or in hand, foot or body baths. American herbalist Susun Weed suggests a black walnut tea soak for fungal toenails or a spritz of tincture for the skin.

A revived Appalachian use, led by Alabama herbalist Phyllis Light, is using the black husks to treat hypothyroidism or goitre. Matthew Wood has confirmed this in hundreds of cases, and calls black walnut *a superlative remedy for hypothyroid*.

While most former uses are now forgotten, walnut's value as an anti-diarrhoeal, insecticide and a dye remains current. Two of the many older virtues, those for skin inflammations and sweating, remain in the 'official' European pharmacopoeia for walnut today.

Modern research

Walnut is often known as 'brain food', and modern research shows why: it increases seratonin levels in the brain (2011). Walnuts as a nutritious food source improved learning and memory function (in rats using maze tests), but also prove a satisfying food in weight-reduction diets. Walnuts in a controlled diet reduced the effects of metabolic syndrome, which is a precursor of diabetes and cardiovascular disease (2012).

A sample of 200 people in a US study (2002) established a positive link between walnut intake and reduced levels of coronary heart disease, with the walnut sample showing lowered blood cholesterol and weight.

Forced-swimming tests in mice (2013) with and without walnut in the diet found that the walnut sample had an anti-fatigue action. This reinforces folk usage of walnuts as a sustaining, easily carried or gathered walking food.

Walnuts are linked to prevention of neurodegenerative disease by maintaining brain health through increasing age (2014a). Another study (2014b) demonstrated improvement in memory deficits and learning skills in mice with induced Alzheimer's disease.

It can be concluded that the benefit/risk assessment for Juglans regia leaves preparations is positive for use in therapeutical dosages in specific conditions of the mild superficial inflammatory conditions of skin and in excessive perspiration of hands and feet.
– European Medicines Agency (2013)

Harvesting walnuts
The green nuts are harvested while the shells inside the husks are still soft for pickling or for making tincture or nocino, a green walnut liqueur. The leaves can be picked any time while they are green, and the ripe nuts are harvested in the autumn.

Muhammara
This Middle eastern walnut spread is traditionally served with pita bread. Mix in a food processor to make a coarse paste: 1 cup **walnuts**, ½ cup **breadcrumbs**, 3 large **roasted red peppers**, 1 teaspoon **cumin**, 2 tablespoons **pomegranate molasses** (or honey), 2 tablespoons **lemon juice**, ½ teaspoon **salt** and 3 tablespoons **extra virgin olive oil.**

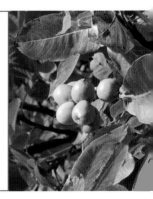

Wild carrot *Daucus carota*, ssp. *carota*

Apiaceae (Umbelliferae) Carrot family

Description: Biennial, to 1m (3ft); fine-leaved, delicate; central florets often red-purple within white umbel; long, fine-cut bracts, which turn upwards, forming a distinctive ball ('bird's nest'); short hairs; stem ridged, unmarked; seeds small, bristly.

Habitat: Grassland, roadsides, wasteland, especially with dry soils.

Distribution: Common in east and south of British Isles, less so upland areas of central Wales and Scotland; naturalised in North America, where it is usually named Queen Anne's lace.

Related species: Cultivated carrot (*D. carota* ssp. *sativus*) is the familiar orange vegetable, with dense green leaves, sometimes seen wild as an escape; sea carrot (*D. carota* ssp. *gummifer*) is local to southern British coasts.

Parts used: Roots, leaves, seeds.

Wild carrot is a tough and beautiful umbellifer that has made the amazing transition from central Asian weed to worldwide food crop. Common on our roadsides, wild carrot can readily be distinguished from its poisonous cousin the hemlock and used medicinally, for urinary tract, reproductive and skincare benefit.

In midsummer the massed white umbels of wild carrot lining the wayside look delicate and 'lacy'. But why the plant should be called Queen Anne's lace – the old British name and now the most frequently used North American name – is something of a mystery.

There are at least three contending Queen Annes and one Saint Anne, and in each case there is a drop or more of blood involved (especially in the case of Anne Boleyn, whose head was cut off). But the elusive historical truth is less important than the visual mnemonic: 'wild carrot' has lacy flowers with pink or purple florets in the centre.

The name and symbol no doubt helped countryfolk of old to distinguish the medicinal and nutritious wild carrot from its deadly poisonous cousin the hemlock (*Conium maculatum*). The two plants have an overlapping wayside habitat and similar British and American distribution; indeed, they can grow alongside and flower at much the same time. Fortunately, hemlock stems have purple or reddish blotches (the *maculatum* of its scientific name) on the stems, while wild carrot has none. These warning blotches are present even when hemlock is a small seedling.

Use wild carrot for...
The seeds of wild carrot are gathered for medicine-making. These are covered with small bristly hairs, which helps them stick to passing animals or humans. Certainly gardeners know that planting the seeds is fiddly because they adhere in a clump, which is why the seeds are often mixed with sand to separate them out and give control over the sowing distance.

The seeds can be eaten, in teaspoonful doses, but they are easier to digest if taken with a little oil, say hemp seed or olive oil (American herbalist Robin Rose Bennett favours almond butter). The oil helps activate the seeds; indeed, if you are taking carrot roots for their vitamin A or beta-carotene, an oil improves absorbtion. Commercial carrot seed oil is an essential oil distilled from wild carrot seed.

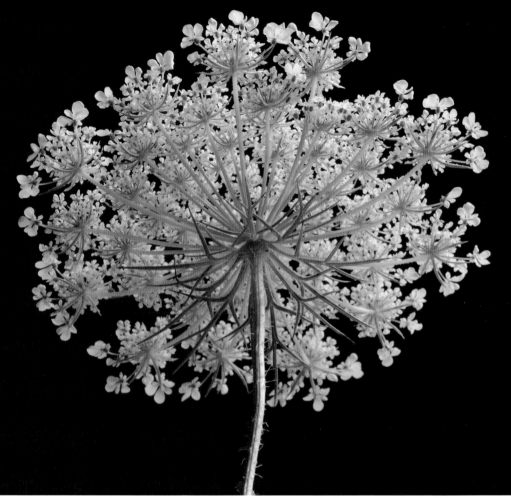

Carrot roots are also macerated in oil for use in skincare products and suntan lotions. Some people may be allergic to these products.

Carrot seeds and roots made into a tea (infusion or decoction respectively) are a traditional diuretic, with a specific action in eliminating urinary stones, and offering relief in urinary tract infections and cystitis. American herbalist Jim Mcdonald likes to combine carrot and goldenrod for urinary issues.

Herbalist Ryan Drum uses chopped carrot leaves or the juice in his gout remedy; he also found that men taking carrot for urinary discomfort had the inadvertent benefit of relief in the initial stages of BPH (benign prostate enlargement) and persistent prostatitis.

Carrot was used to treat worms: Julie's grandmother used grated carrot as a one-day mono-diet for pinworm. This also treats children's threadworms.

Wild carrot flower head, showing the finely divided bracts and hairy stem beneath

Wild carrot seed's double action of relaxing and stimulating unfolds almost entirely on urinary and reproductive functions.
– Holmes (2006)

I like to say that it [carrot] 'helps thread the urine through the kidneys'.
– Wood (1997)

*I regularly prescribe
wild and/or domestic
carrot greens for my
gout patients. ... This
treatment is long-term
(lifetime) to tolerance,
especially for high-
protein diet-induced
gout. The best results
are from finely chopped
leaves in salads or
soups, or leaves juiced
in a wheatgrass juicer.
– Drum (nd)*

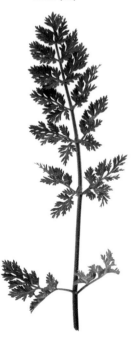

The seed has another familiar use as a 'morning-after' contraceptive. The mechanism seems to be that taking seed extracts prevents implantation of a recently fertilised egg, although stopping the extracts after a period of use may make the woman more fertile. This would explain why carrot seed is variously said to be both abortifacient and reproductive.

Herbalists have a spectrum of views on using carrot seed as a natural birth control, or as a possible strategy (ie taking the seeds and then stopping) for fertilisation. Endocrinal-level research into carrot's action is continuing, and for the time being no firm conclusions can be offered. Accordingly we'd suggest avoiding herbal use of carrot seed during pregnancy (as opposed to eating carrots normally).

Other uses for wild carrot include benefits for asthma sufferers – in ancient Greece carrots were known to calm wheezy horses; as a poultice for cancer sores – a remedy used in Suffolk until about 1920; for help with sugar and tobacco addictions – carry carrots with you and munch when the craving grows; and for a child or infant with diarrhoea a purée of the leaves or root is soothing and replaces lost nutrients. Finally, a carrot flower essence is good for organisation and creativity – it helped us organise our time while writing this book.

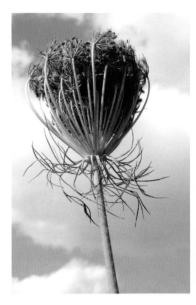

Modern research

Carrot consumption by laboratory rats (2003) modified normal cholesterol absorption and bile acids excretion, and increased antioxidant status. The study found: *these effects could be interesting for* [human] *cardiovascular protection.*

Human subjects drank fresh-squeezed carrot juice (16fl oz daily) for three months (2011a). The finding was that this may protect the cardiovascular system by increasing total antioxidant status and by decreasing lipid peroxidation independent of cardiovascular risk markers.

In a Chinese meta-study in 2014 carrot intake was inversely associated with prostate cancer risk, while the findings of a 2015 meta-study showed an inverse relationship between the consumption of carrots and the risk of gastric cancer.

Carrot juice containing β-carotene or purified β-carotene had antioxidative potential in preventing damage to lymphocyte DNA in smokers (2011b).

Carrot top pesto

Put a couple of handfuls of **young carrot tops** in a saucepan with water to cover and boil for a few minutes, just until they start to wilt. Rinse them under cold water and squeeze dry.

Put in a food processor with 1 clove chopped **garlic**, ½ cup **whole almonds**, with enough **extra virgin olive oil** to blend into a paste (about ½ cup). Add **salt** and **pepper** to taste.

Grated pecorino or other cheese can also be added, as can dill tops and young ground elder leaves.

Carrot seed lozenges

Carrot seeds are covered in small bristles, so are more palatable ground to a powder. Grind 2 tablespoons **carrot seed** in an electric coffee mill or spice grinder. They take longer to grind than you might expect. Strain through a fine sieve to remove any larger bits. You'll end up with just under a tablespoon of powder. Add 1 tablespoon thick **tahini** (sesame paste) and 1 teaspoon of **set honey** (or to taste). Mix until smooth, then roll out with your hands into a thick pencil shape and refrigerate. Cut into a dozen small lozenges, which can be kept in the fridge or freezer, and eat one or two a day.

Carrot top pesto
- gout
- urinary discomfort
- high in potassium
- low libido

Carrot seed lozenges
- sluggish digestion
- tiredness
- convalescence
- low libido

Caution: Be certain of identifying wild carrot before using it. Avoid carrot seeds during pregnancy.

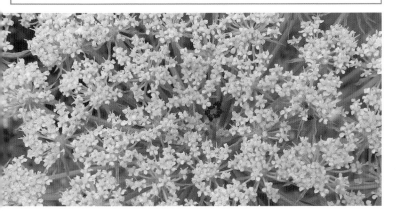

Wild carrot flowers usually have a pink or purple flower in the centre of the umbel

Wild strawberry *Fragaria vesca*

Rosaceae
Rose family

There is nothing quite like the sweet burst of flavour of a tiny wild strawberry, but medicinally the leaves are used to treat digestive and urinary disorders. Modern research is examining strawberry's phytochemical content, with powerful antioxidant potential for treating chronic conditions.

Description: Creeping, 5 to 30cm (3 to 10in) tall, with rooting runners and white flowers, which have rounded edges and no gaps between petals; veined, shiny and pointed trifoliate leaves; fruit resembles a miniature garden strawberry, with pips protruding, sepals turned down.

Habitat: Common on roadsides, hedgebanks, in coppiced woodland or rocky terrain; likes dry, often lime-based soils, eg quarries, railway embankments.

Distribution: Widespread across British Isles, Europe; an introduced alien in North American woods.

Related species: Barren strawberry (*Potentilla sterilis*) is also common, but its fruit is unstrawberry-like. Garden strawberry (*Fragaria x ananassa*) is larger, and may escape to waste ground; Virginia strawberry (*Fragaria virginiana*) is the wild American species, and *F. chiloensis* is the Chilean, once abundant from Chile to Alaska.

Parts used: Berries, leaves, root.

As one of the most recognisable and familiar fruits in the world, the strawberry has been enjoyed for its delicious taste, juiciness and sweet fragrance from Roman times – pips were found in an excavated latrine along Hadrian's Wall – and, from a time before writing, strawberry pips have been dug up at many Mesolithic and Neolithic archaeological sites across Europe.

An early enthusiast and one of the first to mention liking wild strawberries with cream was Cardinal Wolsey (1475–1530). A little later, the physician to James I and VI, Dr William Butler (1535–1618), summarised best the many gustatory tributes paid to this exquisite plant: *Doubtless God could have made a better berry, but doubtless God never did.*

Sugar, to our mind, is optional, and so indeed is cream, if the berries are picked in the sun and eaten. Adding vanilla to the cream will tempt us, while some people soak their berries first in orange juice or kirsch. Matthew's mother sprinkled hers with black pepper.

The origin of the name 'strawberry' is much debated, but one theory can be discounted, namely that it is a berry grown amid straw. This practice arrived centuries after the plant had already been named. More likely its common name is adapted from an Anglo-Saxon term for the berry that 'strews' or spreads itself. The Latin name leaves no doubt: *Fragaria* means sweet-smelling and *vesca* refers to something small.

Unusually, this native wild species did not develop into the strawberry of commerce, but has remained distinct. The strawberry we buy arose from the cross-breeding in the mid-18th century of two introduced species, one from North America and one from South America. Until then garden strawberries were essentially wild strawberries, uprooted and taken into the garden. John Parkinson explained in 1629: *I must also enforme you, that the wilde Strawberry that groweth in the Woods is our Garden Strawberry, but bettered by the soyle and transplanting.*

This was always a limit on strawberry production, with the wild species yielding small-sized fruit in relatively meagre quantities; it tasted wonderful and commanded high prices, but was easily bruised and had a short shelf life. Meeting impatient demand for cheap strawberries was a horticultural holy grail. It needed botanical exploration in the Americas to achieve it.

One notable consumer to make the most of strawberry's availability was the Napoleonic-era *grande dame* Madame Tallien (1773–1836), who reputedly poured 10kg (22lb) of strawberry juice at a time into her bath – but she did not bathe daily.

Meanwhile the wild strawberry has long had its own cultivar, the delicious Alpine strawberry (*F. vesca semperflorens*), or *Fraise des bois* in French.

Use strawberries for...
Eating strawberries is wonderful and indulgent, but is it also good for you? The answer, happily, is yes, whether wild strawberries or cultivated varieties.

Strawberry is alkalising, with high quantities of vitamins and phytochemicals that give it strong antioxidant properties. Its actions are traditionally described as diuretic, laxative and nutritive, and it has been used historically to treat urinary and kidney stones, gout, rheumatism and dysentery, among other conditions.

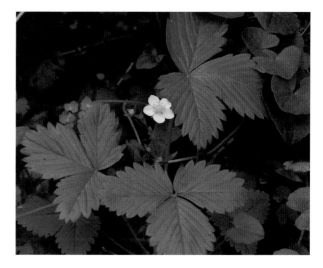

The great botanical systematiser Carl Linnaeus (1707–78) had success with a strawberry fast for his gout, and popularised the cure. Gout is a painful condition caused by excess uric acid, a by-product of purine breakdown, accumulating in the joints and forming crystals. Purines are compounds found in most foods, but particularly in meats and yeast products, including alcohol.

Recent research suggests it is the vitamin C of strawberries that keeps uric acid levels low, thus minimising the risk of gout.

Some researchers, on the other hand, say that strawberries also contain oxalates, which in some people contribute to conditions like stones, urinary tract infections, and indeed gout! The evidence is conflicting, and if you suffer from such conditions

... Mrs Elton, in all her apparatus of happiness, her large bonnet and her basket, was very ready to lead her way in gathering, accepting, or talking. Strawberries, and only strawberries, could now be thought or spoken of. 'The best fruit in England – every body's favourite – always wholesome. ... delicious fruit – only too rich to be eaten much of ... only objections to gathering strawberries the stooping – glaring sun – tired to death – could bear it no longer – must go and sit in the shade.'
– Jane Austen (1816)

The many valuable uses of strawberry have not been entirely understood and utilized.
– Wood (2008)

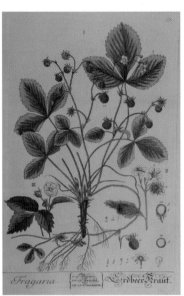

Wild strawberry, painting by Elizabeth Blackwell (1750), courtesy of the Wellcome Library

Fragaria | *Erdbeer Kraut*

Eccentric esculent

Something to munch on when you next eat a strawberry: what we call its fruit or flesh is actually a swollen receptacle, also termed a false or accessory fruit. The real fruit is the achenes, the tiny pips, each containing a single seed, which are dotted on the *outside* of the fleshy receptacle. The cashew shares this quality of the true 'nut' (or pip) being actually the fruit.

Strawberries mislead us: we gobble down the false fruit while obliviously ingesting the real fruit and seeds: it is a brilliant plant trick for spreading itself far and wide! That is, along with the aggressive runners (properly stolons) that enable strawberries to colonise and make a dense ground cover.

and want to treat them through diet and herbs, you are advised to seek practitioner help. If you feel like emulating Linnaeus, taking strawberries as a gout fast should be part of a longer-term controlled diet, including avoiding high-purine foods and alcohol.

The alkalising effect of strawberry underlies its former use in treating tartar (mineralised tooth plaque).

The colour pigments in strawberries (anthocyanins) once served as a rouge to redden light-skinned faces and as medicine for sunburn, burns and minor skin ailments.

Thomas Green's *Universal Herbal* of 1820 says: *It would be unpardonable not to inform our fair readers of these attributes.* At the

same time, it should be noted that some people can suffer an allergic reaction to strawberry on the skin, including urticaria.

The best-known herbal use of strawberry is making an infusion of the leaves, whether using wild-gathered or cultivated forms. Similar to the leaf tea made from its rose family cousins, raspberries or blackberries, strawberry tea is mildly astringent. This astringency underlies its traditional use in relieving diarrhoea and dysentery and settling an over-acid stomach.

The roots as a decoction or tincture are stronger and more 'binding', but are less used than the leaves.

An early English reference to strawberry use is found in The *Old English Herbarium*, written around the year 1000, which recommends the juice of the wild plant, mixed with honey and pepper, for sufferers from asthma or abdominal pain.

The French herbalist Jean Palaiseul (1973) suggests that chilblains in winter can be prevented by rubbing the affected parts in summer with crushed strawberries, and using poultices of pulped strawberries overnight. A messy, if fragrant remedy!

Modern research

There has been much research into strawberries as functional foods, ie valuing it for its nutrients but also as a source of phytochemicals with antioxidant power. For example, an influential paper by Hannum (2004) suggests that strawberry phytochemicals like ellagic acid and various flavonoids inhibit LDL-cholesterol oxidation and plaque stability and decrease tendency to thrombosis (ie reducing cardiovascular risk).

The same research also found that strawberry phytochemicals attack COX enzymes (ie reduce inflammatory processes), and have anti-cancer effects on tumours and carcinogenesis, with marked benefits for the ageing brain.

Research in 2014 suggests frozen strawberries have greater antioxidant potential than fresh or dried ones, while organically grown berries inhibited colon and breast cancer cells (2006), and Vitamin C had a synergistic action with the other compounds.

Other work (2015) indicates how polyphenols in strawberries are effective in treating 'oxidative stress-driven pathologies', which includes cancers, cardiovascular diseases, type II diabetes, obesity, neurodegenerative diseases and inflammation.

Harvesting wild strawberries is hard work, with lots of bending and scrambling, for what are often tiny fruits, but it is well worth the effort. When you find a precious patch of the ripe red fruit, take a shallow basket and line it with a tea towel, so that the collected berries are not crushing each other too much.

Distilled strawberry water
Set up a saucepan as described on page 17, placing the strawberries around your central bowl in a large saucepan and adding enough water to cover them. Place the lid on upside down, with ice on top, and heat gently. When most of the water containing the strawberries has evaporated and been collected in the bowl, remove the lid and bottle your strawberry water.
Dose: 1 dessertspoon internally as needed to calm the heart.

Strawberry leaf tea
This is best made with the fresh leaves, which being evergreen are available most of the year. For maximum flavour, crush the leaves gently with your hands or with a rolling pin before making the tea.

Use 3 or 4 **strawberry leaves** per mug of **boiling water**, steeped in a teapot for about 5 minutes. Strain as you pour into cups. It will be a pretty light yellow colour, with a delicate and refreshing taste. Try it with lemon added.

Of all the many astringents available I find small doses of this one [strawberry leaf] almost irreplaceable in the treatment of peptic, especially gastric ulcers.
– Barker (2001)

Distilled strawberry water
- eyewash for infections or grit in the eyes
- heart palpitations
- cleaning wounds and ulcers

Strawberry leaf tea
- peptic ulcers
- stomach over-acidity
- diarrhoea

Woundwort

Marsh woundwort, *Stachys palustris;* Hedge woundwort, *S. sylvatica*

**Lamiaceae
Deadnettle family**

Description: Both
main species are
perennials of up to
a metre tall. Marsh
woundwort (*Stachys
palustris*) has spear-
shaped leaves and
pinkish-purple flowers.
Hedge woundwort (*S.
sylvatica*) has nettle-
shaped leaves and dark
reddish-purple flowers,
and smells unpleasant
when crushed.

Habitat: Marsh wound-
wort grows in damp
places; hedge wound-
wort prefers woodland
and shade, and is often
a garden weed.

Distribution: Both are
widely distributed in
Britain and Ireland, and
in much of Europe and
Asia. Marsh woundwort
is also found in parts
of the US and Canada,
where it is considered
a weed.

Related species:
Over 300 species in
the genus worldwide.
Field woundwort, *S.
arvensis*, is a near-
threatened annual
weed on arable land.
Betony, *S. officinalis*, is
a well-known medicinal
plant, common in
England and Wales.
The woolly white *S.
byzantina*, lamb's
ear, is often grown in
gardens.

Parts used: Above-
ground parts. The tuber
of *S. palustris* is edible.

Marsh woundwort and hedge woundwort are, unsurprisingly, useful for treating wounds. They are also an effective remedy for insect bites and stings, an antispasmodic and show promise as cardioprotective and being useful in diabetes.

Also called hedgenettles, woundworts are closely related to the medicinal herb betony (or wood betony), *S. officinalis* syn. *Betonica officinalis*. The Chinese artichoke, *S. affinis*, is similar but is grown for its edible white tubers.

The edible swollen white roots of marsh woundwort are also very tasty as a vegetable, and are smoother and easier to clean. They can be eaten raw, being sweet and crunchy, and are delicious fried in a little butter or oil, having a flavour much like skirret.

John Gerard, writing in 1597, reports how he learnt the use of this herb from a labourer he met in Kent. Gerard was a barber-surgeon of some repute in London, and named the plant Clown's woundwort, because the man in question had 'clownishly' turned down Gerard's expert help and preferred to treat his scythe wound with his own home-made woundwort poultice.

Gerard's plant was almost certainly marsh woundwort, as his woodcut shows the small tubers that form among the roots.

Gerard found in his practice that woundwort worked much faster to heal wounds than the balm he had previously used.

He gives two examples of cases where it rapidly healed otherwise mortal wounds. One gentleman, Mr Edward Cartwright, had been stabbed through the base of the sternum into his lungs, and was dangerously feverish. *With this Clownes experiment and some of my*

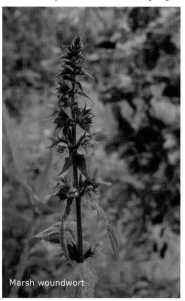
Marsh woundwort

foreknown helpes, Gerard mashed the woundwort with hog's grease and applied it. *By God's permission I perfectly cured* [him] *in a very short time.*

The second case was of a shoemaker's apprentice who had tried to kill himself by stabbing himself through the trachea, in the chest and twice in the abdomen.

Gerard says: *the which mortall wounds, by Gods permission, and the vertues of this herbe, I perfectly cured within twenty daies: for which the name of God be praised.*

Use woundwort for...
On a less dramatic scale, woundwort is a great first aid remedy for minor injuries. Simply crush the leaf in your hands or chew it, then apply. Drinking the tea as well will increase the healing effects. You can also use the tea to soak some gauze and apply it as a fomentation.

A fresh leaf also works well for insect bites and stings, crushed or chewed and rubbed on the bite. Marsh woundwort is more effective than hedge woundwort, but if the latter is all you have to hand it will still help.

Woundwort tea can be beneficial for hay fever and other allergies, as well as for headache and neuralgia. It has similar relaxing effects to betony, well known for being relaxing and protective for the nervous system.

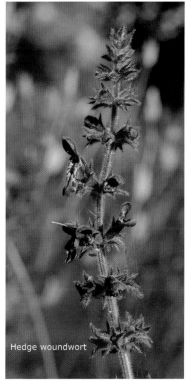

Hedge woundwort

The leaves heerof stamped with Axungia or Hogs grease, and applied unto green wounds in manner of a pultis, doth heale them in such short time & in such absolute maner, that it is hard for any that hath not had the experience thereof to beleeve:
– Gerard (1597)

The stincking Dead Nettles, any of the kinds of them, boyled in wine and drunke, doth wonderfully helpe all inward wounds and hurts, bruises, falls or the like, and are singular good also for the spleene, and the diseases thereof: but especially for the hemorrhoides or piles.
– Parkinson (1640)

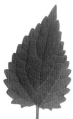

Marsh woundwort leaf

Try it for sleep – have a cup of the tea in the evening. It has been used for cramps (both externally and internally), and also used for gout and pains in the joints. Hand and foot baths using the warm tea are a good way to administer external treatments.

The astringency of both types of woundwort can be used to treat diarrhoea and dysentery. They can be combined with avens, tormentil, silverweed, cinquefoil, agrimony, oak, blackberry leaf and other astringent plants for gum problems, as a mouthwash.

Hedge woundwort leaf

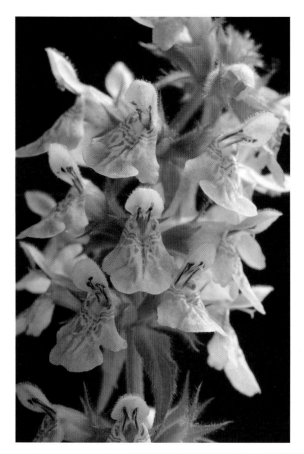

Marsh woundwort can help relax menstrual cramps, and can be combined with black horehound's antispasmodic effects. Woundwort also combines well with the same plant for anxiety and insomnia.

Parkinson mentions woundwort for cancers, a finding that is supported by results of modern research on the essential oil of marsh woundwort.

Modern research
A study of the essential oils of six Mediterranean species of *Stachys* (2009) found that the essential oil of *S. palustris* consisted mainly of carbonylic compounds, showed an anti-free radical effect and a 77% anti-proliferative effect on ACHN cell line (cancer).

Another study (2011) looked at the antibacterial and antifungal properties of the essential oils of 22 different species of *Stachys*. Most of them demonstrated moderate activity against the organisms tested.

Marsh woundwort flowers are beautiful in close-up

Woundwort fresh poultice
- pimples
- cuts & grazes
- insect bites & stings

Woundwort fresh poultice
Crush or chew a leaf or two and apply to insect bites and stings, cuts, grazes and spots. Marsh woundwort is the most effective.

Marsh woundwort roots
The white fleshy roots and tubers are easiest to harvest if you grow your marsh woundwort in a pot sunk into damp ground. In autumn, lift the plant from the pot and harvest the roots / tubers, then replant.

The fresh roots have a raw peanut flavour. When boiled gently so they still have a little crunch, they taste like starchy bean sprouts, very mild and pleasant. Serve with garlic butter, or add to stir fries.

Notes to the text
Recommended reading
Resources
Index

A summer afternoon in
the Lincolnshire Wolds,
with hogweed prominent

Notes to the text

Full citation given in first reference only, thereafter author and page number (or short title if more than one work by that author). Original year of publication is in square brackets; place of publication London unless otherwise stated. For PubMed citations, we give date and reference number (or short title) for follow-up on a search engine. Scientific names of the plants are as given in The Plant List, www.theplantlist.org

Motto [6]: William Coles, *Adam in Eden: Nature's Paradise* (London, 1657) 54; Gabrielle Hatfield, *Memory, Wisdom and Healing* (Stroud, Glos, 1999) 14.

Preface [7]: Charles Dickens, *Nicholas Nickleby* (1839) ch 8; 'undiscovered country': see Robert Macfarlane, *The Wild Places* (2008 [2007] 225; Christopher Hedley, seminar (6 Dec 2014); David Winston, 'The American Extra Pharmacopoeia', www. herbalstudies.net [accessed 21 Sep 2016]; John Ruskin, qtd ES Rohde, *A Garden of Herbs* (Boston MA, 1931) 1.

Introduction [9]: Plantlife, *The Good Verge Guide* (2016).

Harvesting from the wayside [10]: James Green, *The Herbal Medicine-Maker's Handbook: A Home Manual* (Berkeley CA, 2000) 10; Nicholas Culpeper, *Pharmacopoeia Londinensis, Or, The London Dispensatory Further Adorned* (1653) 1–2; anon, *Stiches in Time: The Wayside Flowers & Country Remedies* (Brockhampton, Heref, 2008) 12; Dr John R Christopher, *School of Natural Healing* (Springville UT, 1996 [1976]) viii.

Using your wayside harvest [13]: Christopher Hedley & Non Shaw, *A Herbal Book of Making & Taking* (2016 [1993]) 2.

ALEXANDERS [20]: Geoffrey Grigson, *The Englishman's Flora* (1958) 229; John Parkinson, *Theatrum Botanicum* (1640) 929; William Salmon, *Botanalogica* I (1710) 10; John Aubrey, in *Wiltshire Collections*, ed JE Jackson (1862) 12, cited by Katie Peebles, in *Studies in Medievalism XXVI* (forthcoming, Cambridge, 2017); Columella: www.seedaholic.com [accessed 8 Dec 2015]; RE Randall, *J*

Ecology 91 (2) (2003) 325–40; Culpeper, *Pharm Lon* 19; Covent Garden: Gabrielle Hatfield, *Hatfield's Herbal* (2007) 7; PubMed: (2014) 24924290; (2012) 21902563; (2008) PMC2731181; Anne Pratt, *Haunts of the Wild Flowers* (1866) 310; John Parkinson, *Paradisi in Sole* (1629) 492; *The Syon Abbey Herbal, AD 1517*, ed J Adams & S Forbes (2015) 227.

ASH [24]: overview: Forestry Commission, www.forestrygov.uk [accessed 21 Sep 2016]; 'Betty': *The Guardian*, 22 Apr 2016; biochar: www. carbongold.com [accessed 21 Sep 2016]; John Wesley, *Primitive Physick* (Bristol, 1765 [1747]) 102; Robert Penn, *The Man who Made Things out of Trees* (2015) 7; Oliver Rackham, *The Ash Tree* (Toller Fratrum, Dors, 2014) 8; French herbalist: Jean Palaiseul, *Grandmother's Secrets* (1973 [1972]) 38; William Langham, *The Garden of Health* (1578) 39; Maurice Mességué, *Health Secrets of Plants and Herbs* (1979 [1975]) 40; PubMed: (2014) 24877717; (2015) 24562238; (2010) 20035854; (2004) 15120454; EMA Monograph 239271 (2011).

AVENS [28]: 'antidote': *Hatfield's Herbal* 184; eugenol research: (2011) 1627964; *Ortus Sanitatis*, quoting Plaetarius of Salerno: James T Shipley, *Dictionary of Early English* (Lanham MD, 2014 [1955]) 92; Parkinson, *Theatrum* 138; Henriette Kress, *Practical Herbs* 1 (Helsinki, 2011) 96; David Hoffmann, *Medical Herbalism* (Rochester VT, 2003) 114–17; Sir John Hill, *The Family Herbal* (Bungay, Suff, 1812 [1755]) 19; Edward Baylis, *A New and Compleat Body of Practical Botanic Physic* (1791) 66; www. wildplantforager.com/blog [accessed 22 Sep 2016]; PubMed: (2013) 23738465; (2015) PMC4461949; (2016)

27353564; Palaiseul 39; Julian Barker, *The Medicinal Flora of Britain and Northwestern Europe* (West Wickham, Kent, 2001) 178.

BISTORT [32]: Mrs M Grieve, *The Modern Herbal* (1931) 105; root, snake names: eg Lesley Gordon, *A Country Herbal* (Exeter, 1980) 23; Grigson 247; Turner: Grigson 248; David Blackwell, pers comm, 2014; bistort competitions: eg Stephen Barstow, *Around the World in 80 Plants* (East Meon, Hamp, 2014) 263; Lord Haw Haw, Amundsen: Barstow 260; tanning: Thomas Green, *The Universal Herbal* II (Liverpool, 1820) 376; PubMed: (2014) 24742754; (2016) 26929003; (2008) 18067063; (2015) 26360047; (2011) 21413092; Barker 93.

BLACK HOREHOUND [36]: cattle rejection: Gordon 93; Turner: Grigson 349; Cape use: Ben-Erik Van Wyk et al, *Medicinal Plants of South Africa* (Pretoria, 1997) 54; Richard Lawrence Hool, *Health from British Wild Herbs* (Southport, 1924 [1918]) 5–6; Hoffmann 533; Matthew Wood, *The Earthwise Herbal: Old World Medicinal Plants* (Berkeley CA, 2008) 126–7; Dioscorides: Andrew Chevallier, *Encyclopedia of Herbal Medicine* (2016 [1996]) 176; PubMed: (2010) 20645243; (2008) 18817140; (2003) 15138012; (2014) PMC4099109; John Gerard, *Herball* (1597).

BLACKTHORN [40]: Ötzi: James H Dickson et al, 'The Iceman Reconsidered' (2005), www. scientificamerican.com [accessed 22 Sep 2016]; 'thorn in the flesh': II Cor 12.7; Maj Thomas Weir: Susan Lavender & Anna Franklin, *Herbcraft* (Chieveley, Berks, 1996) 114; 'lady of pearls': *Hatfield's Herbal* 27; Parkinson, *Theatrum* 1034; Palaiseul 286; anon, qtd Hatfield, *Memory* 56; Hill, *Family Herbal* 314; Brooks & Hellier, wine merchants, qtd Roger Phillips, *Wild Food* (1983) 132; *umeboshi*: *The Oxford Companion to Food*, ed Alan Davidson (Oxford, 1999) 726; PubMed: (2009) 20120103; (2014) 24243401; (2013) 23815554; Abbé Kneipp, qtd Palaiseul 286.

BUGLE [44]: Gerard: qtd *Hatfield's Herbal* 46; surgeons: eg Parkinson, *Theatrum* 528; Culpeper, *Pharm Lon* 15; Grigson 354; Langham 99; Parkinson, *Theatrum* 526; Baylis 223–34; William Kemsey, *The British Herbal* (1838), cited in *Hatfield's Herbal* 46–7; harpagide: *Potter's Herbal Cyclopaedia*, ed EM Williamson (Saffron Walden, Ess, 2003) 75; Thomas Green I, 70; PubMed: (2011) 22015320; (2008a) 19478420; (2008b) 18520054.

BUTCHER'S BROOM [48]: Chevallier, *Encyclopedia* (2016) 265; 'knee holly': Langham 111; Parkinson, *Theatrum* 253; rodents: Richard Mabey, *Flora Britannica* (1996) 433; meat trade: *The Encyclopedia of Herbs and Herbalism*, ed Malcolm Stuart (1979) 256; Devon: *Hatfield's Herbal* 52; Christine Herbert, pers comm, 31 Oct 2016; Elizabeth Blackwell, *A Curious Herbal* (1750 German edn of 1739 edn) pl 155; PubMed: (2009) 19620698; (2000) 11152059.

CHICORY [50]: Passover / seder, leaf recipe: Maida Silverman, *A City Herbal* (Woodstock NY, 1997 [1977]) 34–5; Pliny: Lisa Manniche, *An Ancient Egyptian Herbal* (1989) 88; Linnaeus: Silverman 33; names: *Ox Comp Food* 167; Peter Holmes, *The Energetics of Western Herbs*, 2 vols (Boulder CO, 2006 [1989]) I, 449; Camp, poster: Paul Chrystal, *Coffee: A Drink for the Devil* (Stroud, 2016); names: *Ox Comp Food* 167; recurring wartime coffee substitute: Silverman 35; oligofructose: 'Food Unwrapped', Channel 4 TV, 3 Jan 2016, and www.nutriline.org [accessed 4 Jan 2016]; eye issues: HK Bakhru, *Herbs that Heal* (New Delhi, 1990) 66; James Duke, *The Green Pharmacy* (Emmaus PA, 1997) 247; PubMed: (2002) 12860315; (2012)

PMC3372077; (2010) 21694986; (2015) 26151029; Parkinson, *Theatrum* 776.

CRANESBILL [54]: Mrs Grieve 233; Thomas Bartram, *Bartram's Encyclopedia of Herbal Medicine* (1998 [1995]) 134; Culpeper, *Pharm Lon* 18; Salmon I, 229; species numbers: Clive Stace, *Field Flora of the British Isles* (Cambridge, 1999) 316–21; Jim Mcdonald, wild geranium video, 13 Feb 2011; Deni Bown, *Encyclopedia of Herbs & Their Uses* (1995) 288; Holmes II, 797; Michael Moore, *Medicinal Plants of the Mountain West* (Santa Fe NM, 1979) 69; *vrouebossie*, rose geranium: Van Wyk et al, 134; Matthew Wood, *The Earthwise Herbal: New World Medicinal Plants* (Berkeley CA, 2009) 164; PubMed: (2007) 18173115; (2015) 4491959; (2012) 23413565.

CREEPING JENNY & YELLOW LOOSESTRIFE [58]: Parkinson, *Theatrum* 544; Mrs Grieve 549; Turner: Grigson 289; *herbe aux cent maux*: Barker 317; Culpeper, *Pharm Lon* 22; Parkinson, *Theatrum* 555; Hill, *Family Herbal* 204; Dan Bensky & Andrew Gamble, *Chinese Herbal Medicine: Materia Medica* (Seattle WA, 1993 [1986]) 144–5; PubMed: (2002) 12776538; (2013) 263665578.

DAISY [62]: Mrs Pratt, *Haunts* 111; Chaucer, 'The Legend of Good Women' (1385); day's eye: Grigson 400; Milton, 'L'Allegro', l. 75; Shelley, 'The Question', ll. 10–11; Clare, 'The Village Minstrel', ll. 811–12; Hill, *Family Herbal* 107–8; Barker: quote, *bellis* meaning 450; Roman use, soup: Anne McIntyre, *The Complete Floral Healer* (1996) 73; Parkinson, *Theatrum* 532; modern uses: Rachel Corby, *The Medicine Garden* (Preston, 2009) 44; bruisewort: *Hatfield's Herbal* 92; Wesley 67; Elizabeth Blackwell pl 200; Nikki Darrell, pers comm, 27 Jun 2015; Chris Gambatese, pers comm, 17 Jun 2016; PubMed: (2012) 22775421; (2013) 24346069; (1997) 9434600; (2014) 24617777; (2016) 27178360; (2005) 16036165.

FLEABANE [68]: genera: Stace 487–9; Linnaeus: Mrs Grieve 321; Egypt: Manniche 109–10; Parkinson, *Theatrum* 128; Salmon I, 372; Rudolf Koch & Fritz Kredel, *Das Blumenbuchje Zeichungen*, 3 vols (Mainz, 1929–30) III, 215; PubMed: (2012) 02014782; (1992) *Field Mus Nat Hist* 1442; (2014a) 25532299; (2014b) *J Pure App Microbio* 8 (4): 267985.

FORGET-ME-NOT [72]: naming: eg Jack Sanders, *The Secrets of Wildflowers* (Guilford CT, 2014) 121; Gerard: *Hatfield's Herbal* 138; Coleridge, 'The Keepsake', ll. 10–13; DH Lawrence, *Lady Chatterley's Lover* (1928) ch 15; Mrs Grieve 322; Parkinson, *Theatrum* 692; PubMed: (2014) *Acta Phys Plant* 36 (8): 2283–6; (2011) 22462056; (2008) *Chem Nat Comp* 44 (5): 632–3; Parkinson, *Theatrum* 692.

FUMITORY [76]: 'official' (1618): Culpeper, *Pharm Lon* 18; (1996): *British Herbal Pharmacopoeia 1996* (Exeter, 1996) 84; names: Grigson 60; Shakespeare, *King Lear* 4.4.2–6; Mrs Pratt, *Haunts* 74; *Hatfield's Herbal* 142; EMA / HMPC / 576232 / 2010; Mességué 129; Christophe Barnard, seminar, Avignon, 26 Apr 2015; Mrs CF Leyel, *Herbal Delights* (1987 [1937]) 280; Holmes II, 692; Palaiseul 123; India: Elizabeth M Williamson, *Major Herbs of Ayurveda* (Edinburgh, 2002) 150; PubMed: (2012) 23569991; (2014) *J Intercult Ethnopharm* 3 (4): 173–8; (2011) 3371888; Anne Pratt, *Flowering Plants, Grasses, Sedges, and Ferns of Great Britain* 1 (1873) pl 14.

GOLDENROD [80]: Aaron's rod: Grigson 398; *S. odora*, Liberty Tea: Silverman 63; Parkinson, *Theatrum* 543; Gerard: Grigson 399; William Cobbett (1818), qtd Gordon 87; John Muir (1905), qtd Silverman 63; Palaiseul 123; Culpeper, *Pharm Lon* 17; German treatments: Aviva Romm, *Botanical Medicine for Women's Health* (St Louis MO, 2010) 296; tea: Maria Treben, *Health through God's Pharmacy* (Steyr, Austria, 1982) 24; cf green tea: www.herbalremediesadvice.org [accessed 15 Jul 2016]; *BHP 1996* 91; ragweed: Steven Foster & James Duke, *Eastern/Central Medicinal*

Plants and Herbs (New York, 2000) 139; PubMed: (2004) 15638071; (2014) 23872883; (2002) 12467138; (2008) 18380925; (2009) 19827029; (2012) 23137724.

GREATER CELANDINE [84]: Holmes I, 410; Barker 129; Mességué 86; Anne van Arsdall, *Medieval Herbal Remedies* (New York, 2002) 127; Treben 25–6; *Hatfield's Herbal* 155; Langham 128; Pechey 46; Mrs Pratt, *Haunts* 214; PubMed: (1995) 7757387; EMA/HMPC/369801/2009.

GROUND ELDER [87]: Barstow 232; Hill, *Family Herbal* 157; Grelda: Richard Mabey, *Weeds* (2010) 198; Gerard: qtd Pamela Michael, *Edible Plants & Herbs* (2007 [1980]) 107; St Gerard: Bown 229; bishopweed: Grigson 232–3; 'Wildman' Steve Brill & Evelyn Dean, *Identifying and Harvesting Edible and Medicinal Plants* (New York, 2002 [1994]) 260; Mabey, *Weeds* 197; Parkinson, *Theatrum* 944; Tabernaemontanus 1588, qtd in (2009) 19063957; 'all the tastier': John Wright, *Hedgerow* (2010) 101; PubMed: Olga Tovchiga et al, papers, 2012–16; (1987) 24225783; (2007) 17574359.

GROUND IVY [92]: alehoof, gill: Mrs Grieve 442; 'poor name': Grigson 352; Bartram 207–8; *BHP 1996* 95; Hildegard: www.whisperingearth.co.uk [accessed 28 Sep 2016]; Langham 8; 'recent survey': Henriette Kress, *Practical Herbs 2* (Helsinki, 2013) 76–9; Parkinson, *Theatrum* 677; PubMed: (2011) 3218471; (2006) 16530364; (2013) 24477256; (2014) 24850617.

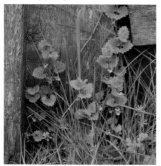

GYPSYWORT [96]: Lyte: qtd Grigson 342–3; Barker 383; Constantine Samuel Rafinesque, *Medical Flora* (1828): see www.henriettes-herb.com [accessed 28 Sep 2016]; Holmes II, 555; Hoffmann 463; PubMed: (2006) 16150466; (1994) 8135877; (2013) 3719484; (2008) 18083068.

HEATHERS [99]: genera: Stace 193–4; George Buchanan, qtd in DC Watts, *Dictionary of Plant Lore* (Burlington MA, 2007) 188; Mrs Pratt, *Haunts* 249–50; Scottish uses: Tess Darwin, *The Scots Herbal* (Edinburgh, 1996) 106–9, and William Milliken & Sam Bridgewater, *Flora Celtica* (Edinburgh, 2013) passim; honey: Milliken & Bridgewater 72–3; Leyden: qtd anon [Elizabeth Kent], *Flora Domestica* (1831) 200; ale/wine: ibid. 58–60; moorland tea: Darwin 108; Koch & Kredel, III, 210; Matthiolus, Clusius: Parkinson, *Theatrum* 1486; PubMed: (2014) 25550074; (2013) 24383325; (2010) 19827032; (2011) 22181981; Dr R Spittal, 'The Heather Bell' (nd), qtd GP Morris & NP Willis, *The Prose and Poetry of England and America* (New York, 1845) 540, www.electricscotland.com [accessed 21 Oct 2016].

HERB ROBERT [104]: redness: Palaiseul 96; Rupert: Barker 212; Robert, Robin Goodfellow: Grigson 114–17, and Katherine Kear, *Flower Wisdom* (2000) 153, 155–6; South Africa: Van Wyk et al, 134; Pechey 118–19; red-water fever, Ireland: David E Allen & Gabrielle Hatfield, *Medicinal Plants in Folk Tradtion* (Portland OR, 2004) 175–6; PubMed: (2010) 21046015; (2004) 15165415; (2012) *Med. Chem. Res.* 21 (5): 601–15; (2014) 3274083; Mrs Pratt, *Haunts* 41; Chevallier 216.

HOGWEED [108]: 'commonest': M Blamey, R & A Fitter, *The Wild Flora of Britain and Ireland* (1977) 180; Heracles/Hercules: Stuart 201; giant hogweed: eg Mabey, *Weeds* (2010) 228–33; French uses: Cathy Skipper, pers comm, 10 Nov 2015; Wood, *Earthwise*:

New World 188; PubMed: (2008) *Planta Med* 74 – PF18; (2013) 23541934; (2014) 24697288; (2010) 20657619; (2006) 16504434; Roger Phillips, *Wild Food* (1983) 50; buds: Mina Said-Allsopp, pers comm, 9 Jan 2016.

LESSER CELANDINE [112]: Wordsworth: Miranda Seymour, *A Brief History of Thyme* (2002) 18; DH Lawrence, *Sons and Lovers* (1913) ch 6; names: Grigson 50; 'broom handle': Seymour 18; Parkinson, *Theatrum* 618–19; Pechey 47; Parkinson 289–90; Culpeper, *Pharm Lon* 17; 'as in other cases': Allen & Hatfield 83; causes: Barker 119; PubMed: (2015) 25729484.

MOUSE-EAR HAWKWEED [116]: Hill, *Family Herbal* 236; William Curtis, *Flora Londinensis* 2 (1835 [1778]) 274; Parkinson, *Theatrum* 790; *BHP 1983*: Bartram 298; Leo Hartley Grindon, *The Manchester Flora* (1859) 304; expectorant: Hoffmann 512; Pechey 162; Barker 498; New South Wales: www.weeds.dpi.nsw.au [accessed 4 Oct 2016]; PubMed: EMA/HMPC/68034/2013; (2011) *Open Life Sci* 6 (3): 397–404; (2010) 21054887; (2009) 3274148; Chevallier 220.

NAVELWORT [120]: Parkinson, *Theatrum* 741–2; Mrs Grieve 455; names: Grigson 200; Gerard: Mrs Pratt, *Haunts* 192; Culpeper, *Pharm Lon* 25; Sarah Raven, *Wild Flowers* (2011) 100; Miles Irving, *The Forager Handbook* (2009) 294; Barker 16; Bach: www.bachessenceproducers.com [accessed 30 Sep 2016]; Pechey 168; PubMed (2012) 22672636; Van Arsdall 170.

OX-EYE DAISY [124]: Grigson 405–6; gools: www.hikersnotebook.net [accessed 26 Sep 2016]; dermatitis: PubMed (1999) 10439521; www.extension.colostate.edu [accessed 26 Sep 2016]; Pechey 69; Salmon I, 289; Thomas Green I, 294; Hill, *Family Herbal* 107; Mabey, *Flora Britannica* 373; PubMed: (2015) 26121329.

PINE [128]: John Evelyn, *Sylva* (1664) I, 242; Pechey 188; Julia Lawless, *The Encyclopaedia of Essential Oils* (Shaftesbury, 1992) 157; drovers:

Hatfield's Herbal 268; Matthiolus: Parkinson, *Paradisi* 608; Linnaeus, flour: Laura Mason, *Pine* (2013) 153, 156; sanitoria, asthma: Nikki Darrell, *Conversations with Plants* (Cork, 2014) I, 176; 'truism': Parkinson, *Theatrum* 1538; Peter Conway, *Tree Medicine* (2001) 234–5; Keats, 'Ode to Psyche' (1819) l. 53; Charlotte du Cann, *52 Flowers that Changed My World* (Uig, Isle of Lewis, 2012) 172; Michael Moore, *Medicinal Plants of the Desert and Canyon West* (Santa Fe NM, 1989) 89; Euell Gibbons, *Stalking the Healthful Herbs* (New York, 1966) 122, qtd Mason 156; Wood, *Earthwise: New World* 269; Crispin Van de Pas, *Hortus Floridus* (Arnhem, 1614) pl 78; PubMed: (2009a) 2794845; (2005a) 15752644; (2000) 10857921; (2002) 11996210; (2005b) 16028975; (2009b) *Food & Bio Proc* 88 (2–3): 247–52.

PRIMROSE & COWSLIP [134]: Chevallier 256; Plantlife survey, 9 Jun 2015, www.plantlife.org [accessed 3 Aug 2016]; St Peter's keys: Philippa Back, *The Illustrated Herbal* (1987) 48; Freya, overpicking: McIntyre 181; W Strehlow & G Hertzka, *Hildegard of Bingen's Medicine* (Santa Fe NM, 1988) 82; Treben 22; Parkinson, *Paradisi* 247; George Eliot, *Mill on the Floss* (1860), bk 1, ch 7; Pechey 60; Milton: Colonial Dames of America, *Herbs and Herb Lore of Colonial America* (New York, 1995 [1970]) 48; Germany, 'official': NG Bisset & M Wichtl, *Herbal Drugs and Phytopharmaceuticals* (Stuttgart & Boca Raton FL, 2001 [1994]) 389, 391; Wesley 123; Saskia Marjoram: www.saskiasfloweressences.com [accessed 26 Sep 2016]; PubMed: (2012) PMC 3318187; (1994) 23195935.

PURPLE LOOSESTRIFE [139]: 'reliable drama': Raven 316; 'long purples': Grigson 209; 'iron hard': Sybil Marshall, *Fenland Chronicle* (Cambridge, 1980 [1967]) 196; 'purple plague': Timothy Lee Scott, *Invasive Plant Medicine* (Rochester VT, 2010) 255–60; Salmon 604, 652; '2.7 million seeds': www.seagrant.umn.edu [accessed 4 Oct 2016]; '$45m': www.refugeassociation.org [accessed 4 Oct 2016]; Mcdonald: www.herbcraft.

org [accessed 4 Oct 2016]; Parkinson, *Theatrum* 547; Anna Parkinson, pers comm, 28 May 2013; Mrs Grieve 497; PubMed: (2010) 20554008; (2012) 22829057; (2015) 25985768; (2005) 15975734.

ROWAN [144]: names: Grigson 186–7; 'rowan': *Hatfield's Herbal* 296; James VI & I, *Demonologie* (Edinburgh, 1598) IV, 3; tanning, dyeing: Mrs Grieve 69; parasorbic acid: Irving 285; PubMed: (2008) 18819524; (2010) 21195756; 'The Laidly Worm', qtd Wright 77; Rev J Evans, *Letters Written through a Tour of North Wales* (1798) 112; Alys Fowler, *The Thrifty Forager* (2011) 172.

SANICLE [148]: 'molecular': Raven, 25; ancient woodland: Oliver Rackham, *Woodlands* (2006) 325; 'Celui qui…': qtd WT Fernie, *Herbal Simples* (Philadelphia, 1895) 508; Grigson 224; Parkinson, *Theatrum* 534; Elizabeth Blackwell pl 63; Hool 28; PubMed: (1999) 10441789; (1996) 8769089; (2013) 23770053; Jethro Kloss, *Back to Eden* (New York, 1939) 309; Wood, *Earthwise: Old World* 461, attrib to Peter Holmes.

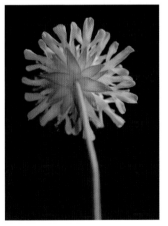

SCABIOUS [152]: genera: www.theplantlist.org [accessed 23 Sep 2015]; Knaut: Mrs Grieve 721; 'rough stalks': Mabey, *Flora Britannica* 363; devil's bit name: Grigson 386–7, Barker 385; devil's 'envy': *Grete Herball* (1526), in Grigson 387; plague: Marcus Harrison,

Plants and the Plague (Lostwithiel, Corn, 2015) 197–201; Parkinson, *Theatrum* 490; Culpeper: Mrs Grieve 722; Hill, *Family Herbal* 306; Stuart 268; Holmes I, 233; PubMed: (2015) 25841374; (2012) 22492499; (2010) 2984435.

SEA BUCKTHORN [157]: migrant birds: Mabey, *Flora Britannica* 233; HCA Vogel, *The Nature Doctor* (1989 [1952]) 387; Parkinson, *Theatrum* 1008; elder health: eg Barker 246; 'New Nordic': www.washingtonpost.com, 25 Jul 2016 [accessed 10 Oct 2016]; 'Siberian pineapple': *Sea Buckthorn*, ed V Singh & H Kallio (New Delhi, 2003) 486; John Wilkes, ed, *Encylopaedia Londinensis* 10 (1811) 192; PubMed: (2012) 3317027; (2006) 16968106; (2011) 21960663; (2009) 19425187; (2003) 12854177; (2013) 23096237; (2016) *Afr J Biotech* 15 (5): 118–24; Wright 156; harvesting: eg Irving 290; ice cream sauce: noted Davidson 708.

SILVERWEED, TORMENTIL & CINQUEFOIL [162]: tormentil names: Grigson 161; 'austere': Hill, *Family Herbal* 342; silverweed names: Grigson 159; argentina, goosewort: Stuart 245; prince's feathers: Zöe Hawes, *Wild Drugs* (2010) 70; Alexander Carmichael: radix4roots.blogspot (2011) [accessed 7 Oct 2016]; Ray: Grigson 160; Wright 78; cinquefoil: Mrs Grieve 316; cinquefoil names: Grigson 162–3; crampwort: Holmes II, 795; Vogel 218; Mrs Leyel, *Cinquefoil: Herbs to Quicken the Five Senses* (1957) 9; Parkinson, *Theatrum* 399; 'sisters': Palaiseul 257; Pechey 236; PubMed: (2009) 19857087; (2014a) 4202341; (2003) 12913771; (2014b) 25483225; (2008) 18664379; (2011) 20677176; Barker 180.

SOWTHISTLE [166]: genera: Stace 452–3, 475; Margaret Roberts, *Margaret Roberts' Book of Herbs* (Johannesburg, 1983) 120; Barstow 167; Arthur Lee Jacobson: www.arthurleej.com [accessed 2 Oct 2016]; Pliny: Mabey, *Flora Britannica* 365; Popeye, worldwide uses: Irving 158; passover, Five Boro: Brill & Dean 201–2; Ray: qtd Grigson 322; warts, latex: Allen

& Hatfield 282; Parkinson, *Theatrum* 807; opium: Brill & Dean 202; Nepal: Narayan P Manandhar, *Plants and People of Nepal* (Portland OR, 2002) 433; elder medicine in China: Silverman 151; PubMed: (2002) 12716920; (2012) 3292812; (2011) 3305921.

SPHAGNUM MOSS [176]: Mrs Grieve 554; British / Irish species: British Bryological Society, *Mosses and Liverworts of Britain and Ireland: A Field Guide* (2010) 276–310; Cathcart, poem: Peter Ayres, *Field Bryology* 110 (2013): www.rbg-web2.rbge.org.uk [accessed 1 Oct 2016]; Nelson Coon, *Using Wild and Wayside Plants* (New York, 1980 [1957]) 84–5.

SPEEDWELL [170]: Mrs Grieve 831; species: Stace 414–18; 'victory': Grieve 831; Roberts 62; Parkinson, *Theatrum* 552; Francke: Bown 368; Pechey 222; *thé d'Europe*: Barker 408; Leclerc, poor man's tea, eyebright, whooping cough: *Hatfield's Herbal* 326; cholesterol, Roman compliment, priest: Treben 40–1; brooklime like scurvy grass: Raven 292; Wright 128; PubMed: (2013) 23142555; (1985) 4021513; (2014) 24892270.

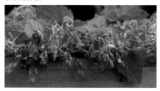

SWEET CHESTNUT [178]: Evelyn I, ch 8; Bartram 109; Pechey 53; Bach remedy: Conway 153; bud: Joe Rozencwajg, *Dynamic Gemmotherapy* (New Plymouth NZ, 2008) 39–40; *The Times* (London) 22 Aug 2015; PubMed: Quave et al (2015) 4546677.

THISTLE [182]: 'Scotch thistle': Mabey, *Flora Britannica* 455; Scott: www.nrscotland.gov.uk [accessed 9 Oct 2016]; Irving 147; Hill, *Family Herbal* 337; silymarin: Holmes I, 196; Barker 483; Katrina Blair, *The Wild Wisdom of Weeds* (White River Junction VT, 2014) 311–31; Wesley 80, 117; Blair 321–2; Matthew Alfs (2014), *Medical Herbalism* 17 (2): 8–15.

VALERIAN [187]: odour: Antony Dweck, in Peter J Houghton (ed), *Valerian: The Genus Valeriana* (Amsterdam, 1997) 2; 'phu', kesso root, jatamansi: Mrs Grieve 824, 828–9; Gerard, *Herball* (1636 edn) 1078; Robert Thornton, *A New Family Herbal* (1810) 35; Pied Piper, eg Doug Elliott, *Wild Roots: A Forager's Guide* (Rochester VT, 1995) 87; Fabius Columna: Seymour 119; Pechey 240; John Hill, *The Virtues of Wild Valerian in Nervous Disorders* (1772 [1758]); *U.S. Pharmacopoeia*: Roy Upton et al, *Valerian Root* (American Herbal Pharmacopoeia, Santa Cruz CA, 1999) 2; *BHP 1996* 176; 'nauseous': Grieve 827; Gustave Flaubert, *Madame Bovary* (1857): qtd Seymour 119; Parkinson, *Theatrum* 124–5; 7Song, seminar, Avignon, 28 Apr 2015; 150 compounds: Upton 8; Barker 431.

VIOLETS [192]: 'dog': Grigson 79; Macer: qtd *Hatfield's Herbal* 336; Leigh Hunt, *The Indicator* (1820); Horace: qtd Bown 370; Romans: Barker 251; Richard Surflet, *A Countrie Farme* (1600); Lightfoot: qtd *Hatfield's Herbal* 336; Hill, *Family Herbal* 362; Maria Sybilla Merian, *Erucam ortus…* (Amstelaedami, 1718) pt 2, pl 1; *Hamlet* 1.3.7–10; ionones: www.boisdejasmin.com [accessed 29 Sep 2016]; Violetta: Bown 370; 'pectoral': Palaiseul 306; 'official': *BHP 1996* 178; Nicholas Culpeper, *The English Physician Enlarged* (1814 [1652]) 337; Askham: qtd Mrs Grieve 835; Duke, *Green Pharmacy* 446; South Africa: Roberts 45; Salerno: qtd Palaiseul 306; Langham 663; PubMed: (1995) 7703226; (2010a) 20564026; (2010b) 20580652; (2008) 18081258; (2011) 22242426; (2014) 25763239; (2015) 25954025.

WALNUT [198]: Jupiter: Stuart 208; Parkinson, *Theatrum* 1413–14; Thomas Fuller, *The History of the Worthies of England* (1682 [1662]) 76; Evelyn I, ch 9; JC Loudon, *Arboretum et Fruticetum Britannicum* (1838); Roger Deakin, *Wildwood: A Journey through Trees* (2007) 317; brain / *charmarghz*: Davidson 833; Coles: Mrs Grieve 844; Culpeper, *Pharm Lon* 11–12; Willis: Harrison 223; Langham 666; Pliny, hair recipe: Stuart 208; Susun Weed, video

[last accessed 30 Oct 2016]; Wood, *Earthwise: New World* 208; PubMed: (2011) 22048906; (2012) 23756586; (2002) 11983340; (2013) 24396383; (2014a) 24500933; (2014b) 25024344; EMA / HMPC / 346740 / 2011, 26.

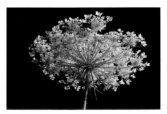

WILD CARROT [202]: Forgotten Herbs blog, July 2016; Robin Rose Bennett: blog, 1 July 2012; Holmes II, 574; Matthew Wood, *The Book of Herbal Wisdom* (Berkeley CA, 1997) 230; Ryan Drum: blog, nd; Jim Mcdonald: blog, 13 Feb 2006; bird's nest: Elliott 75; Suffolk: Gabrielle Hatfield, *Country Remedies* (Woodbridge, Suffolk, 1994) 24; PubMed: (2003) 14569406; (2011a) 3192732; (2014) 24519559; (2015) 26819805; (2011b) 3259297; Duke, *Green Pharmacy* 400; Saskia Marjoram: www.saskiasfloweressences.com [accessed 26 Sep 2016].

WILD STRAWBERRY [206]: Hadrian's Wall: *Hatfield's Herbal* 331; Wolsey, Mme Tallien: Ernest Small, *Top 100 Food Plants* (Ottawa, 2009) 493; Dr Butler: Izaak Walton, *Compleat Angler* (1653) pt I, ch 5; Parkinson, *Paradisi* 526; Linnaeus: Richard Pulteney, *A General View of the Writings of Linnaeus* (1805) 478–80; Jane Austen, *Emma* (1816) ch 36; Wood, *Earthwise: Old World* 261; Elizabeth Blackwell pl 77; Thomas Green I, 574; Van Arsdall 168; Parkinson, *Theatrum* 758–9; Hill, *Family Herbal* 329; Palaiseul 294; PubMed: (2004) 15077879; (2014) 24345049; (2006) 16478244; (2015) 25803191; Barker 180.

WOUNDWORT [210]: Gerard: Wood, *Earthwise: Old World* 471; Parkinson, *Theatrum* 609; blog: monica.wilde.com, 16 Aug 2015 [accessed 5 Oct 2016]; PubMed: (2009) 22339365; (2011) *Phytochem Lett* 4 (4): 448–53.

Recommended reading

Barker, Julian. *The Medicinal Flora of Britain & Northwestern Europe: A Field Guide*. West Wickham, Kent, 2001

Barstow, Stephen. *Around the World in 80 Plants*. East Meon, Hampshire, 2014.

Bartram, Thomas. *Bartram's Encyclopedia of Herbal Medicine*. London, 1998 [1995]

Blair, Katrina. *The Wild Wisdom of Weeds: 13 Essential Plants for Human Survival*. White River Junction, VT, 2014

Bruton-Seal, Julie & Matthew Seal. *Hedgerow Medicine*. Ludlow, Shropshire, 2008

_____ *The Herbalist's Bible*. Ludlow, Shropshire, 2014

Campbell, Ffyona. *The Hunter-Gatherer Way: Putting Back the Apple*. South Hams, Dorset, 2014 [2012]

Cech, Richo. *Making Plant Medicine*, 4th edn. Williams, OR, 2016 [2000]

Chevallier, Andrew. *The Encyclopedia of Herbal Medicine*, 2nd edn. London, 2016 [1996]

_____ *Herbal Remedies*. London, 2007

Coon, Nelson. *Using Wild and Wayside Plants*. New York, 1980 [1957]

Gordon, Lesley. *A Country Herbal*. London, 1980

Green, James. *The Herbal Medicine-Maker's Handbook: A Home Manual*. Berkeley, CA, 2002

Grieve, Mrs M, ed. and introd. Mrs CF Leyel. *A Modern Herbal*. London, 1998 [1931]; online at www.botanical.com

Grigson, Geoffrey. *The Englishman's Flora*. London, 1975 [1958]

Harrap, Simon. *Harrap's Wild Flowers: A Field Guide to the Wild Flowers of Britain & Ireland*. London, 2013

Harrison, Marcus. *Plants and The Plague: The Herbal Frontline*. Lostwithiel, Cornwall, 2015

Hatfield, Gabrielle. *Memory, Wisdom and Healing: The History of Domestic Plant Medicine*. Stroud, Gloucestershire, 1999

_____ *Hatfield's Herbal*. London, 2007

Hedley, Christopher & Non Shaw. *Herbal Remedies: A Practical Beginner's Guide to Making Effective Remedies in the Kitchen*. Bath, 2002 (1996)

_____ *A Herbal Book of Making & Taking*. London, 2016 [1993]

Kress, Henriette. *Practical Herbs*. Helsinki, Finland: vol. 1, 2011; vol. 2, 2013

Mabey, Richard. *Flora Britannica*. London, 1996

_____ *Weeds: How Vagabond Plants Gatecrashed Civilisation and Changed the Way We Think About Nature*. London, 2010

Masé, Guido. *The Wild Medicine Solution: Healing with Aromatic, Bitter, and Tonic Plants*. Rochester, VT, 2013

McIntyre, Anne. *The Complete Floral Healer*. London, 1996

Milliken, William & Sam Bridgewater. *Flora Celtica: Plants and People in Scotland*. Edinburgh, 2013

O'Ceirin, Cyril & Kit. *Wild and Free: Cooking from Nature*. Dublin, 1978

Palaiseul, Jean. *Grandmother's Secrets: Her Green Guide to Health from Plants*. London, 1973 [1972]

Phillips, Roger. *Wild Food*. London, 1983

Pienaar, Antoinette. *The Griqua's Apprentice: Ancient Healing Arts of the Karoo*. Trans. Catherine Knox. Cape Town, 2009

Plantlife. *The Good Verge Guide: A Different Approach to Managing Our Waysides and Verges*. London, 2016

Pole, Sebastian. *Cleanse, Nurture, Restore with Herbal Tea*. London, 2016

Rackham, Oliver. *The Illustrated History of the Countryside*. London, 2003 [1986]

Rohde, Eleanour Sinclair. *A Garden of Herbs*. Boston, MA, 1921; online at archive.org

Scott, Timothy Lee. *Invasive Plant Medicine: The Ecological Benefits and Healing Abilities of Invasives*. Rochester, VT, 2010

Silverman, Maida. *A City Herbal: Lore, Legend, & Uses of Common Weeds*, 3rd edn. Woodstock, NY, 1997 [1977]

Tobyn, Graeme, Alison Denham & Margaret Whitelegg. *The Western Herbal Tradition: 2000 Years of Medicinal Plant Knowledge*. Edinburgh, 2011

Waller, Pip. *The Domestic Alchemist: 501 Herbal Recipes for Home, Health & Happiness*. Lewes, East Sussex, 2015

Wood, Matthew. *The Earthwise Herbal: A Complete Guide to Old World Medicinal Plants*. Berkeley, CA, 2008

_____ *The Earthwise Herbal: A Complete Guide to New World Medicinal Plants*. Berkeley, CA, 2009

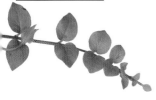

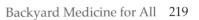

Resources

Finding a herbal practitioner

To find a qualified herbalist near you, contact the professional associations listed below, or check with your local health shop or complementary therapy clinic.

UK

Association of Master Herbalists (AMH) www. associationofmasterherbalists.co.uk

Ayurvedic Practitioners Association (APA) www.apa.uk.com

College of Practitioners of Phytotherapy (CPP) www.phytotherapists.org

International Register of Consultant Herbalists and Homeopaths (IRCH) www.irch.org

National Institute of Medical Herbalists (NIMH) www.nimh.org.uk

United Register of Herbal Practitioners (URHP) www.urhp.com

USA

American Botanical Council (ABC) www.abc.herbalgram.org

American Herbalists' Guild (AHG) www.americanherbalistsguild.com

Workshops

Hedgerow Medicine www.hedgerowmedicine.com The authors' website, offering workshops, short courses; see also closed Facebook group *Forgotten Herbs*, which we moderate.

Suppliers

You can find most of what you need in grocery, kitchen and hardware stores. Here are a few suppliers who carry some of the harder-to-source supplies you might want.

Al-Ambiq www.al-ambiq.com Beautiful hand-made copper stills from Portugal.

G Baldwin & Co www.baldwins.co.uk Mail order and shop: brown glass bottles, lanolin, beeswax; also dried herbs, essential oils.

Lakeland Ltd www.lakeland.co.uk Mail order and shops: jam- and jelly-making supplies, kitchen equipment.

Just Botanics www.justbotanics.co.uk Mail order for tinctures, oils, dried herbs, gums, resins, powders and empty capsules.

The London Teapot Company www.chatsford.com Mail order, manufacturer: Chatsford teapots with basket strainers for loose teas.

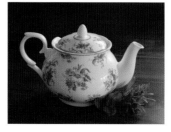

Plant information

Henriette Kress www.henriettesherbal.com Well-respected herbal information website, with complete texts of many older herbals.

Michael Moore www.swsbm.com Inspirational website of the late American herbalist (1941–2009), featuring distance learning.

The Herb Society www.herbsociety.org.uk Promotes interest in all aspects of herbal use, publishes *Herbs* magazine.

Plantlife International www.plantlife.org.uk The wild-plant conservation charity.

State of the World's Plants sotwp_2016 Pioneering report by Kew Royal Botanic Gardens.

The Wildlife Trusts www.wildlifetrusts.org Local groups, nature reserves.

Seeds and plants

Many plant nurseries sell wildflower seeds and plants. Two of our favourites are:

Poyntzfield Herb Nursery www.poyntzfieldherbs.co.uk For beautifully packed seeds and plants.

British Wild Flower Plants www.wildflowers.co.uk Largest supplier of British native plants.

Index

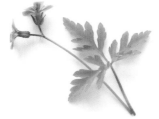

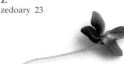

The authors

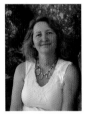

JULIE BRUTON-SEAL is a practising medical herbalist, iridologist and cranio-sacral therapist. A Fellow of the Association of Master Herbalists (AMH), she is also a writer, photographer, artist and graphic designer. Julie co-authored the vegetarian cookbook *Vegetarian Masterpieces* (1988).

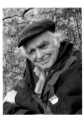

MATTHEW SEAL has worked as an editor and writer in books, magazines and newspapers for over forty years, in both the UK and South Africa. He is author of *Survive and Thrive in the New South Africa* (2000), and was the founder of the Professional Editors' Group there in 1993. He has served as the publications director of the Society for Editors and Proofreaders (SfEP).

Julie and Matthew teach courses and workshops in herbal medicine. For more information, visit the Facebook pages for their books and see their website: www.hedgerowmedicine.com

Other books by Julie and Matthew:

Hedgerow Medicine

Harvest wild plants and weeds and make your own remedies from the hedgerow. A practical guide to 50 common plants, telling you exactly what to do with them and how to use them, with recipes for each plant.

Published in North America as *Backyard Medicine.*

My absolute herbal inspiration nowadays being Julie and Matthew's wonderful book Hedgerow Medicine, *which to my mind is the best home-use British herbal that has ever been written – such a beautiful, inspiring and empowering book!*

Rose Titchiner, flower essence maker and author

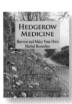

Kitchen Medicine

You have a pharmacy at your fingertips in your own pantry, and this practical book shows you how to use herbs, spices, fruits, vegetables, oils, vinegars and other familiar kitchen items to treat common ailments.

This is the best book I have ever seen on this subject and I just want to buy it for everyone I know! It is a great resource, an inspiration, a thing of great beauty and healing. Everyone should have a copy in their kitchens!

Permaculture Magazine

Make Your Own Aphrodisiacs

This attractive book is full of delicious recipes for romance, and is sumptuously illustrated. From ashwagandha to yohimbe via chocolate, roses, horny goat weed and more, this is a guide to herbs that really work as aphrodisiacs. Many of these herbs are also rejuvenating tonics.

It was published in North America as *Aphrodisia: homemade potions to make love more likely, more pleasurable and more possible.*

This would make a lovely Christmas present or indeed a fun, but informative, gift for lovers of both plants and people at any time of the year. I liked its small size – handy for the bedroom – and the rich, colourful pictures lend themselves very well to romance and the love of life in general.

The Herbalist

The Herbalist's Bible
John Parkinson's Lost Classic Rediscovered

A selection from and commentary on the biggest and best herbal ever written in English, John Parkinson's magnum opus, the largely forgotten *Theatrum Botanicum* or *Theater of Plants* (1640). Herbalist to Charles I, Parkinson took 50 years to write this book, and his experience comes through clearly in the Vertues (medicinal uses) for the chosen plants. Julie and Matthew add their own comments and illustrations.

… a fascinating fusion of old and new.
The English Gardener